# Table of Contents

# Introduction

Keto diet is one of the prominent and demand diets nowadays. It allows to eat delicious and nutritious meals without any calories restrictions and at the same time - lose weight and burn fat. Nevertheless, there is a food list which helps to clarify what food is better to avoid while following Keto diet.

The fundamental principle of the Keto diet is "to get rid of fat - you should eat fat and restrict carb consuming". Commonly the energy source for the body is carbs. Nevertheless, according to the Keto diet rule, our body starts using fat as a fuel source of energy. It causes the elevated Ketones in the bloodstream. This process is called ketosis.

The diet has an extremely huge amount of benefits. Besides weight loss, Keto diet refines skin health, hormonal balance, and improve memory and cognitive function. In some cases, the Keto diet helps to maintain the steady-state health and fight with Type 2 diabetes.

Keto diet has four different variations. It is significant to determine the right Keto diet type according to your health and medical appointments.

Let's find out four types of Keto diet.

The first one and the most popular is *Standard Ketogenic Diet (SKD)*. This diet assumes consuming of 75 % fats, 5 % carbohydrates, and 20 % proteins.

Next one is *High Protein Keto Diet (HPKD)*. Usually, this type is recommended for sportsmen or people with an extremely active lifestyle. According to this type it is allowed to eat 35 % proteins, 60 % fat, and 5 % carbs.

The third one is *Cyclical Ketogenic Diet (CKD)* It includes the mixture of standard Ketogenic diet (5-6 days) and then low-carb days for 1-2 days; after this repeat the circle. This diet is recommended for people with the extremely high need in carbs.

The last type of Keto diet is *Targeted Ketogenic Diet (TKD)*. It is recommended for athletes. The directions for the diet are: consuming maximum 25 grams of net carbs one hour before the gym.

Keto diet involves the consumption of not more than 25 grams of carbohydrates per day and only 7 grams of them have to be net carbs.

In an era of lack of time and a busy lifestyle, it is vital to eat right balanced food. Thanks to instant pot it became accessible to save time and cook not only useful and nutritious but also delicious food.

This book includes 125 various recipes for everyday meal and for special events. All the recipes are created for 2 servings that allows to follow diet together and save time in counting the right amount of ingredients. Here you will find tasty breakfast recipes, gorgeous ideas for lunchtime and side dishes, simple but incredible recipes of main dishes and desserts. Everything you need to start following the Keto diet is your desire and inspiration!

# Breakfast Recipes

### Soft-Boiled Eggs
*Prep time: 5 minutes | Cooking time: 3 minutes | Servings: 2*

**Ingredients:**
- 4 eggs
- ¾ teaspoon dried thyme
- ¾ teaspoon chili flakes

**Directions:**

Pour 1 cup of water in the instant pot bowl and add eggs. Close the lid of the instant pot and seal it. Chose the "Steam" program (High Pressure) and cook the eggs for 3 minutes. Then remove the cooked eggs from the instant pot and place them in the icy water. Let them chill for 1 minute. Peel the eggs and cut them into the halves. Sprinkle the egg halves with the chili flakes and dried thyme and serve immediately!

**Nutrition value/serving:** calories 262, fat 19.43, fiber 0.4, carbs 2.6, protein 18.09


### Spinach Frittata
*Prep time: 5 minutes | Cooking time: 10 minutes | Servings: 2*

**Ingredients:**
- 2 eggs
- 1 cup spinach, chopped
- 1 teaspoon cream cheese
- 2/3 teaspoon ground black pepper
- ½ teaspoon butter

**Directions:**

Grease the instant pot pan with butter. Beat the eggs in the separated bowl and whisk them well. After this, add cream cheese and ground black pepper. Stir it gently. Place the chopped spinach in the greased pan and add the whisked eggs. Pour 1 cup of water in the instant pot. Place the trivet in the instant pot and transfer the egg mixture pan on the trivet. Close the instant pot and set the "Manual" (High Pressure) program and cook frittata for 5 minutes then make naturally release for 5 minutes more and serve the breakfast.

**Nutrition value/serving:** calories 151, fat 11.42, fiber 0.6, carbs 2.26, protein 9.68

# Breakfast Meatballs

*Prep time: 10 minutes | Cooking time: 15 minutes | Servings: 2*

**Ingredients:**

- 10 oz chicken fillet
- 1 egg
- 1 tablespoon coconut flour
- ¾ teaspoon salt
- ¾ teaspoon paprika
- ¾ teaspoon chili pepper
- ¾ teaspoon ground black pepper
- ½ teaspoon butter
- ¾ teaspoon dried dill

**Directions:**

Chop the chicken fillet into the tiny pieces. Mix up together the coconut flour, paprika, chili pepper, ground black pepper, and dried dill. Stir the mixture gently. After this, combine together the chicken and coconut flour mixture. Stir it well and beat the egg in the mixture. Mix it up until you get homogenous mass. Make the medium meatballs from the mixture. Grease the instant pot pan with the butter and place the meatballs. Add ¼ cup of water and close the instant pot. Set the "Manual" program (High pressure) for 8 minutes. After this, make quick release and chill the meatballs little.

**Nutrition value/serving:** calories 296, fat 17.58, fiber 1.1, carbs 4.94, protein 30.19


# Tender Chicken Breast with Coconut Milk

*Prep time: 10 minutes | Cooking time: 15 minutes | Servings: 2*

**Ingredients:**

- 12 oz chicken breast, skinless, boneless
- ½ teaspoon salt
- ½ teaspoon white pepper
- ½ teaspoon ground black pepper
- ½ cup coconut milk
- ½ teaspoon paprika
- 1 teaspoon dried parsley

**Directions:**

Mix up together salt, white pepper, ground black pepper, paprika, and dried parsley. Rub the chicken breast with the spice mixture generously. After this, place the chicken breast in the instant pot bowl. Add coconut milk and close the lid. Set the "Poultry" program and cook the chicken for 8 minutes. After this, make the naturally release for 5 minutes. Slice the chicken breast and sprinkle with the remaining coconut milk sauce from instant pot. Serve it!

**Nutrition value/serving:** calories 335, fat 18.6, fiber 1.7, carbs 4, protein 37.6

## Crunchy Bacon Strips

*Prep time: 5 minutes | Cooking time: 5 minutes | Servings: 2*

**Ingredients:**
- 2 eggs, beaten
- 6 oz bacon, sliced
- ¾ teaspoon chili pepper

**Directions:**
Sprinkle the sliced bacon with the chili pepper and place in the instant pot bowl. Add the beaten eggs and close the lid. Cook the meal on "Manual" program for 4 minutes. Make the natural release and serve the meal immediately.

**Nutrition value/serving:** calories 524, fat 39.9, fiber 0.1, carbs 1.8, protein 37.1

## Morning Burrito Bowl

*Prep time: 8 minutes | Cooking time: 12 minutes | Servings: 2*

**Ingredients:**
- 10 oz chicken fillet
- 5 oz avocado, cored
- 1 teaspoon butter
- ¼ teaspoon salt
- ½ teaspoon ground black pepper
- 1 cucumber, chopped
- 3 tablespoons coconut milk

**Directions:**
Cut the chicken fillet into the strips and sprinkle with the salt and ground black pepper. Place the chicken in the instant pot bowl and add butter and coconut milk. Stir it gently and close the lid. Set the "Poultry" program and cook it for 7 minutes (naturally release for 5 minutes). Meanwhile, slice avocado and place it into the serving bowls. Add chopped cucumber. Add the cooked chicken strips and serve the meal immediately.

**Nutrition value/serving:** calories 386, fat 20.1, fiber 2.4, carbs 8.3, protein 42.9

# Breakfast Casserole

*Prep time: 7 minutes* | *Cooking time: 9 minutes* | *Servings: 2*

**Ingredients:**

- 2 eggs
- ¼ cup full-fat cream
- ¼ teaspoon salt
- 3 oz asparagus, chopped
- 2 oz tomato
- 3 oz Parmesan, shredded
- 1 teaspoon butter
- 1 teaspoon ground paprika

**Directions:**

Slice the tomato into thick pieces. Grease the instant pot pan with the butter. Beat the eggs in the bowl, add salt, and ground paprika. Whisk the eggs well. After this, add chopped asparagus and tomato. Pour the mixture into the instant pot pan and sprinkle over with the shredded cheese. Pour 1 cup of the water in the instant pot. Place the trivet inside the appliance. Then place the pan with the egg mixture on the trivet and close the lid. Cook the meal on "Manual" program (High pressure) for 4 minutes. Then make naturally release for 5 minutes.

**Nutrition value/serving:** calories 437, fat 37.7, fiber 1.2, carbs 6.3, protein 21.7

# Egg Cups

*Prep time: 5 minutes* | *Cooking time: 15 minutes* | *Servings: 2*

**Ingredients:**

- 2 eggs
- ¼ cup cream cheese
- 3 oz bacon, fried, chopped
- ¾ teaspoon butter
- ¼ teaspoon ground black pepper

**Directions:**

Pour 1 cup of water in the instant pot bowl. Beat the eggs in the bowl and combine together with the cream cheese. Whisk the mixture. Add ground black pepper. Then place the chopped bacon into the mason jars. Add the whisked egg mixture and butter. Cover the mason jars with the foil. Place the trivet in the instant pot and transfer the mason jars on the trivet. Close the instant pot lid and set the "Steam". Cook the meal for 10 minutes. After this, make the quick release (QR) for 5 minutes. Chill the egg cups little and serve!

**Nutrition value/serving:** calories 407, fat 33.7, fiber 0.1, carbs 1.9, protein 23.5

## Morning Cups
*Prep time: 6 minutes | Cooking time: 3 minutes | Servings: 2*

### Ingredients:
- 3 eggs, beaten
- ¼ cup spinach
- 2 oz green pepper, chopped
- 1 tablespoon coconut milk
- ¼ teaspoon salt
- ½ teaspoon ground white pepper
- ¾ teaspoon butter

### Directions:
Chop the spinach and then blend it with the help of the hand blender. Mix up together the blended spinach and beaten eggs. Whisk the mixture. Add coconut milk, ground white pepper, green pepper, and butter. Stir it gently. Pour the water in the instant pot. Place the trivet in the instant pot. After this, pour the egg mixture into the small cups and transfer them on the trivet. Close the lid and set "Manual" program (High Pressure). Cook the morning cups for 3 minutes. Make a quick release. Serve the meal immediately!

**Nutrition value/serving:** calories 132, fat 9.9, fiber 0.9, carbs 2.7, protein 8.9

## Quiche
*Prep time: 10 minutes | Cooking time: 6 minutes | Servings: 2*

### Ingredients:
- 3 eggs, beaten
- 1 tablespoon coconut flour
- 4 oz Parmesan, shredded
- 5 oz prawns, peeled
- 1 tablespoon cream cheese
- ¼ cup spinach
- ½ teaspoon hot chili pepper
- 1 tablespoon butter

### Directions:
Whisk the eggs and coconut flour together. Chop the prawns roughly and add in the egg mixture. After this, chop the spinach and add in the egg mixture too. Add butter and hot chili pepper. After this, add cream cheer and mix up the mixture very carefully. Place the mixture into the quiche pan. Sprinkle the mixture with Parmesan over. Then transfer the pan in the instant pot and close the lid. Set the "Manual" program and cook quiche for 6 minutes. Then make the quick release and chill the meal little. Cut the quiche into halves and serve!

**Nutrition value/serving:** calories 446, fat 27.8, fiber 1.6, carbs 6.5, protein 43.7

## Stuffed Eggs with Bacon

*Prep time: 5 minutes | Cooking time: 5 minutes | Servings: 2*

**Ingredients:**

- 2 eggs
- 4 oz fried bacon
- 1 tablespoon butter
- ¾ teaspoon salt
- ¾ teaspoon ground black pepper
- ¾ teaspoon fresh parsley

**Directions:**

Pour 1 cup of water in the instant pot bowl and add eggs. Seal the instant pot lid. Set the "Steam" program and cook the eggs for 5 minutes. Then make a quick release. Meanwhile, melt the butter and mix it up with the salt, ground black pepper, and fresh parsley. Chill the cooked eggs and cut them into the halves. Remove the egg yolks and add them into the butter mixture. Stir carefully until homogenous. Then fill the egg whites with the butter mixture and serve the eggs warm.

**Nutrition value/serving:** calories 423, fat 33.9, fiber 0.2, carbs 1.7, protein 26.7

## Chicken Roll

*Prep time: 8 minutes | Cooking time: 12 minutes | Servings: 2*

**Ingredients:**

- 4 oz bacon, sliced
- 9 oz chicken breast, skinless, boneless
- 1 tablespoon butter
- ½ teaspoon ground black pepper
- ¼ teaspoon chili flakes
- ½ teaspoon white pepper
- ¼ teaspoon thyme
- 3 oz white mushrooms, chopped

**Directions:**

Beat the chicken breast well with the help of the kitchen hammer to get the tender piece. Then sprinkle the chicken breast with the ground black pepper, white pepper, and thyme. Place in the center of the chicken breast chopped white mushrooms and butter. Roll up the chicken breast and wrap it in the sliced bacon. Wrap the chicken roll in the foil. Set the instant pot mode "Poultry" and place the chicken roll in the instant pot bowl. Cook the chicken roll for 12 minutes. Then make naturally pressure release. Slice the chicken roll and serve!

**Nutrition value/serving:** calories 518, fat 32.8, fiber 0.9, carbs 3.5, protein 49.6

# Egg Bites

*Prep time:* 5 minutes | *Cooking time:* 7 minutes | *Servings:* 2

**Ingredients:**
- 4 eggs
- 4 oz Parmesan, shredded
- 1 teaspoon butter
- ¾ teaspoon salt

**Directions:**
Grease the instant pot pan with the butter generously. Then beat the eggs in the bowl and whisk well. Add salt and shredded Parmesan. Stir the eggs gently and transfer into the greased instant pot pan. Place the pan into the instant pot and close the lid. Cook the meal on "Manual" mode (High pressure - QR) for 5 minutes to get the solid eggs. Then remove the pan with eggs from the instant pot and cut the egg meal into the medium bites. Serve the meal hot!

**Nutrition value/serving:** calories 325, fat 22.8, fiber 0, carbs 2.7, protein 29.3

# Cheese Omelet

*Prep time:* 5 minutes | *Cooking time:* 3 minutes | *Servings:* 2

**Ingredients:**
- 2 eggs
- 1/3 cup full-fat cream
- ¾ teaspoon chili flakes
- ½ teaspoon butter
- 2 oz Cheddar cheese, shredded

**Directions:**
Beat the eggs in the bowl and whisk them carefully. Add full-fat cream, chili flakes, and stir the mixture. After this, grease the pan with the butter and pour the egg mixture inside. Sprinkle the egg mixture with the shredded cheese. Pour ½ cup of water in the instant pot bowl and place the trivet. Transfer the pan on the trivet and close the lid. Cook omelet on "Manual" mode for 4 minutes (Naturally release). Serve the cooked meal immediately!

**Nutrition value/serving:** calories 211, fat 17, fiber 0, carbs 2, protein 12.9

## Breakfast Porridge
*Prep time: 5 minutes | Cooking time: 3 minutes | Servings: 2*

**Ingredients:**
- ¾ cup shredded coconut
- 3 tablespoons coconut milk
- 3 tablespoons water
- 1 teaspoon coconut flour
- 1 tablespoon psyllium husk
- ¾ teaspoon vanilla extract
- ¾ teaspoon ground cinnamon

**Directions:**
Place the shredded coconut in the instant pot and toast it for 2-3 minutes at "Saute" mode. Stir it time to time. Then add water and coconut milk and mix up until homogenous. Add coconut flour, psyllium husk, vanilla extract, and ground cinnamon. Stir again. Close the lid. Set the "High pressure" mode with a timer to 0. When the time is up, make the naturally release for 9 minutes. Open the lid and transfer the cook

**Nutrition value/serving:** calories 212, fat 15.5, fiber 18.2, carbs 24.4, protein 1.7

## Pork Bites
*Prep time: 10 minutes | Cooking time: 20 minutes | Servings: 2*

**Ingredients:**
- 10 oz pork loin
- 1 teaspoon rosemary
- ¼ cup water
- 1 oz onion, chopped
- ½ garlic clove
- ½ teaspoon ground black pepper
- ½ teaspoon salt

**Directions:**
Chop the pork loin into the medium pieces. Sprinkle the meat with the rosemary, chopped, onion, salt, and ground black pepper. Chop the garlic clove and add it in the meat. Mix up the meat mixture with the help of the hands. Pour water in the instant pot bowl and add meat mixture. Close the lid and set the "Meat/Stew" mode. Cook the meal for 20 minutes. Then chill the meat until warm and serve!

**Nutrition value/serving:** calories 353, fat 19.9, fiber 0.7, carbs 2.3, protein 39

# Bacon Muffins

*Prep time: 5 minutes | **Cooking time:** 9 minutes | **Servings:** 2*

**Ingredients:**
- 2 tablespoons coconut flour
- 1 egg, beaten
- 3 oz bacon, chopped fried
- 1 teaspoon dill
- ¼ teaspoon salt
- 1 tablespoon cream cheese

**Directions:**
Whisk the beaten egg with the help of the hand whisker. Stir the coconut flour into the whisked egg and add dill, salt, and cream cheese. Mix up the mixture until homogenous. Pour the mixture into the muffin molds and top with the fried bacon. Pour 1 cup of water in the instant pot and place trivet. Transfer the muffin molds on the trivet and close the instant pot lid. Set the "manual" mode and cook the muffins for 4 minutes. Make naturally pressure release for 5 minutes.

**Nutrition value/serving:** calories 310, fat 22.5, fiber 3.1, carbs 6.2, protein 20

# Light Stuffed Green Peppers

*Prep time: 6 minutes | **Cooking time:** 8 minutes | **Servings:** 2*

**Ingredients:**
- 2 green peppers
- 2 eggs
- 1 oz Parmesan, shredded
- ¼ teaspoon butter
- ¼ teaspoon ground black pepper

**Directions:**
Cut the green peppers into the halves and remove the seeds. After this, beat the eggs into the bowl and whisk gently. Add shredded cheese and ground black pepper. Put the small piece of the butter in every green pepper half. Then add the whisked eggs. Place the foil into the instant pot bowl and transfer the peppers there. Close the lid and cook the peppers on "Manual Mode" High pressure for 3 minutes. Make naturally pressure release for 5 minutes.

**Nutrition value/serving:** calories 137, fat 8.1, fiber 2.1, carbs 6.5, protein 11.2

## Creamy Boiled Eggs

*Prep time: 10 minutes | Cooking time: 5 minutes | Servings: 2*

### Ingredients:

- 4 eggs
- 1 oz avocado, peeled
- ¾ teaspoon chili flakes
- 1 teaspoon butter, melted
- ¼ teaspoon fresh dill, chopped
- 3 oz lettuce

### Directions:

Pour 1 cup of water in the instant pot bowl and add eggs. Set the "Steam" mode on your instant pot and cook the eggs for 5 minutes (QR). Meanwhile, mix up together the melted butter, fresh dill, and chili flakes. Churn the mixture. When the eggs are cooked transfer them in icy water for 3 minutes. After this, peel the eggs. Place the eggs in the blender and blend until smooth. Add the churned butter mixture and blend it for 30 seconds more. Fill the lettuce leaves with the egg mixture and serve immediately!

**Nutrition value/serving:** calories 178, fat 13.5, fiber 1.3, carbs 3.3, protein 11.6

## Stuffed Avocado Boats

*Prep time: 10 minutes | Cooking time: 7 minutes | Servings: 2*

### Ingredients:

- 1 avocado
- 4 oz shrimps
- 1 tablespoon cream cheese
- ¾ teaspoon salt
- ¼ teaspoon dried oregano
- 1 garlic clove
- ½ teaspoon butter

### Directions:

Cut the avocado into the halves and remove the pip. Peel the shrimps and chop them roughly. Sprinkle the shrimps with the salt and dried oregano. Chop the garlic clove and add in avocado mixture. Then put the small piece of butter in every avocado half. Add shrimp mixture and cream cheese. Wrap the avocado halves into the foil and place in the instant pot. Set the "Stew" mode and cook the avocado boats for 7 minutes (QR). Unwrap avocado halves and chill them for 1-2 minutes.

**Nutrition value/serving:** calories 301, fat 23.3, fiber 6.8, carbs 10.3, protein 15.3

# Keto Breakfast Sandwich

*Prep time: 10 minutes | Cooking time: 10 minutes | Servings: 2*

**Ingredients:**

- 4 oz lettuce leaves
- 8 oz chicken fillet
- 1 tablespoon butter
- 1 oz onion, chopped
- 1 oz lemon
- ¼ teaspoon hot chili pepper
- 2 teaspoons full-fat cream
- ¼ cup water

**Directions:**

Dice the chicken fillet and sprinkle it with the chopped onion, and hot chili pepper. Squeeze the lemon juice over the poultry. Transfer the poultry into the instant pot; add water and butter. Close the lid and cook the chicken on "Poultry" mode for 10 minutes. When the chicken is cooked – place it on the lettuce leaves to make the medium sandwiches. Sprinkle the sandwiches with the chicken gravy.

**Nutrition value/serving:** calories 287, fat 14.5, fiber 1.1, carbs 4.5, protein 33.5

# Breakfast Chicken Hash

*Prep time: 15 minutes | Cooking time: 7 minutes | Servings: 2*

**Ingredients:**

- 1 oz celery stalk
- 1 onion, chopped
- ¾ cup water
- 1 teaspoon coconut milk
- ½ teaspoon butter
- ½ teaspoon ground black pepper
- ½ teaspoon rosemary
- 10 oz chicken fillet, diced

**Directions:**

Set the "Stew" mode and toss the butter in the instant pot. When the butter is melted – add the diced chicken. Sprinkle it with the ground black pepper, chopped onion, and add water. Chop the celery stalk and add in the chicken. Add coconut milk. Close the lid and cook the meal for 7 minutes (High pressure). Make the natural pressure release for 10 minutes.

**Nutrition value/serving:** calories 310, fat 12.2, fiber 1.7, carbs 6.2, protein 41.9

# Lemon Salmon Fillet

*Prep time:* *7 minutes* | *Cooking time:* *8 minutes* | *Servings:* *2*

**Ingredients:**

- 1 teaspoon butter
- ½ teaspoon dried thyme
- ¾ teaspoon nutmeg
- ¾ teaspoon garlic powder
- 10 oz salmon fillet
- 1 oz lemon, sliced
- 4 tablespoons almond milk

**Directions:**

Rub the salmon fillet with the garlic powder, dried thyme, and nutmeg. Grease the instant pot pan with the butter. Place the salmon fillet in the instant pot pan and top it with the sliced lemon. Add almond milk and cover the pan with the foil. Pour 1 cup of water in the instant pot and place the trivet. Put the pan on the trivet and close the instant pot lid. Set the "Stew" mode and cook the meal for 8 minutes. Serve the meal with remaining gravy from instant pot pan.

**Nutrition value/serving:** calories 286, fat 18.2, fiber 1.4, carbs 4.3, protein 28.6


# Coconut Milk Prawns

*Prep time:* *5 minutes* | *Cooking time:* *5 minutes* | *Servings:* *2*

**Ingredients:**

- 8 oz prawns, peeled
- 1/3 cup coconut milk
- ½ teaspoon garlic powder
- 1 teaspoon butter
- ½ teaspoon hot chili pepper

**Directions:**

Set the "Meat'Stew" mode on instant pot Toss butter in the instant pot bowl and add prawns. Sprinkle the prawns with the garlic powder and hot chili pepper. Cook for 1 minute. Add coconut milk and close the lid. Cook the prawns for 3 minutes on "Meat/Stew" mode. Serve the meal hot!

**Nutrition value/serving:** calories 247, fat 13.4, fiber 1, carbs 4.6, protein 26.9

# Eggplant Kebob

*Prep time: 7 minutes | Cooking time: 10 minutes | Servings: 2*

**Ingredients:**

- 1 eggplant
- 1 green pepper
- 7 oz chicken breast, skinless, boneless
- 1 tablespoon coconut oil
- ½ teaspoon ground black pepper

**Directions:**

Chop the eggplant and green pepper into the cubes. Chop the chicken breast into the cubes. Sprinkle all the ingredients with the coconut oil and ground black pepper String the vegetables and poultry on the wooden skewers. Place the kebobs on the trivet and transfer the trivet in the instant pot. Add ½ cup of water in the instant pot bowl and close the lid. Cook the meal on "Manual" (High Pressure) mode for 5 minutes. Then make naturally pressure release for 5 minutes. Serve the kebobs immediately!

**Nutrition value/serving:** calories 226, fat 9.5, fiber 9.2, carbs 16.6, protein 20.8

# Lunch Recipes

### Lasagna with Zucchini
*Prep time: 10 minutes | Cooking time: 12 minutes | Servings: 2*

Ingredients:
- 4 oz zucchini
- 8 oz ground beef
- 1 tablespoon cream cheese
- 1 oz Parmesan cheese, shredded
- ½ tomato

Directions:

Slice the zucchini. Set the "Saute" mode at the instant pot and add ground beef. Chop the tomato and add in the meat. Saute the meat for 6 minutes, stir it from time to time. When the meat is cooked – remove it from the instant pot. Take the springform pan and place the layer of the sliced zucchini. Then add the layer of the ground beef. Sprinkle the layer with the small amount of the shredded cheese. Then put the layer of the zucchini and repeat the same with all the ingredients. Top the lasagna with the remaining cheese. Pour 1 cup of water in the instant pot. Place the steam rack. Transfer the lasagna on the steam rack and close the lid. Cook the meal on "Steam" mode for 6 minutes (QR). Serve the meal warm.

Nutrition value/serving: calories 286, fat 12, fiber 0.8, carbs 3.1, protein 40.2

### Keto Stuffed Peppers
*Prep time: 10 minutes | Cooking time: 15 minutes | Servings: 2*

Ingredients:
- 2 green peppers
- 5 oz ground beef
- 1 garlic clove, chopped
- ¼ teaspoon salt
- ¾ teaspoon ground black pepper
- 2 teaspoon cream cheese
- 1 oz white onion, chopped
- ½ cup water

Directions:

Wash the green peppers carefully and cut off the top parts. Discard all the seeds from inside. After this, mix up together the chopped garlic, salt, ground black pepper, and chopped onion. Stir it well. Fill the peppers with the ground beef mixture. Top every pepper with the cream cheese. Pour water in the instant pot and add the steam rack. Place the peppers on the steam rack and close the instant pot lid and seal it. Set the "Manual" mode and put the timer on 9 minutes. Make natural release then (appx. 5 minutes). Serve the meal immediately!

Nutrition value/serving: calories 177, fat 5.8, fiber 2.6, carbs 7.9, protein 23.1

## Cauliflower Cream Soup

*Prep time: 5 minutes | Cooking time: 8 minutes | Servings: 2*

**Ingredients:**
- 1 cup chicken stock
- 1 teaspoon butter
- 1 tablespoon full-fat cream
- ½ teaspoon paprika
- 2 oz bacon, chopped, fried
- 1 oz Parmesan, shredded
- 4 oz cauliflower, chopped

**Directions:**
Pour the chicken stock in the instant pot bowl. Add butter, full-fat cream, paprika, and cauliflower. Close the lid and seal it. Set the "Manual" mode and turn on the timer on 8 minutes (High pressure). Make quick release then. Use the hand blender to make the liquid smooth. Add fried bacon and Parmesan. Stir the soup and serve!

**Nutrition value/serving:** calories 246, fat 18.1, fiber 1.6, carbs 4.9, protein 16.8

## Shredded Beef

*Prep time: 10 minutes | Cooking time: 35 minutes | Servings: 2*

**Ingredients:**
- 9 oz beef tenderloin
- ¾ cup water
- 1 onion, peeled
- ½ teaspoon salt
- ½ teaspoon hot chili pepper
- 1 tablespoon butter

**Directions:**
Chop the beef tenderloin and place in the instant pot. Add water, onion, salt, hot chili pepper, and butter. Lock the instant pot lid and set "Manual" mode (High Pressure) for 25 minutes. Then make natural pressure release for 10 minutes. Remove the meat from the instant pot and shred it with the help of the fork. Add little bit gravy and serve!

**Nutrition value/serving:** calories 336, fat 17.5, fiber 1.2, carbs 5.3, protein 37.6

## Meatball Stew

*Prep time: 15 minutes | Cooking time: 10 minutes | Servings: 2*

**Ingredients:**

- 4 oz eggplant
- 8 oz ground beef
- ½ teaspoon white pepper
- ½ teaspoon ground paprika
- 1 tablespoon full-fat cream
- ¾ cup water
- ½ teaspoon turmeric
- 1 teaspoon coconut flour
- ¾ onion, chopped

**Directions:**

Peel the eggplants and chop them. Mix up together the ground beef, white pepper, ground paprika, turmeric, coconut flour, and chopped onion in the separated bowl. Then make the small meatballs. Freeze them for 10 minutes. Place the meatballs in the instant pot bowl. Add chopped eggplants and water. Lock the instant pot lid and set "Manual" mode (High Pressure) for 10 minutes. Then make a quick release. Transfer the cooked stew in the bowls and serve!

**Nutrition value/serving:** calories 255, fat 7.8, fiber 3.8, carbs 9.2, protein 35.8

## Garlic Salmon

*Prep time: 7 minutes | Cooking time: 8 minutes | Servings: 2*

**Ingredients:**

- 2 garlic cloves
- ¼ teaspoon garlic powder
- 1 tablespoon fresh dill, chopped
- 1/3 teaspoon salt
- 1 teaspoon paprika
- 10 oz salmon fillet
- 2 tablespoons cream
- 1 teaspoon butter

**Directions:**

Mix up together the garlic powder, chopped fresh dill, salt, and paprika. Rub the salmon fillet with the spice mixture generously. Then peel the garlic cloves and crush them. Place the salmon fillet on the foil and sprinkle with the butter, cream, and add the crushed garlic. Wrap the salmon in the foil. Pour 1 cup of water in the instant pot and add the steamer rack. Place the salmon on the steam rack and lock the instant pot lid. Set the "Steam" mode and cook the salmon for 8 minutes. Unwrap the cooked salmon and serve!

**Nutrition value/serving:** calories 225, fat 11.6, fiber 0.7, carbs 3.1, protein 28.3

## Ropa Vieja

*Prep time: 5 minutes | Cooking time: 50 minutes | Servings: 2*

**Ingredients:**
- 11 oz chuck roast
- ½ white onion, sliced
- 2 oz green pepper
- ½ teaspoon dried rosemary
- 1 teaspoon smoked paprika
- ¼ teaspoon ground cloves
- 1 bay leaf
- 1 teaspoon garlic powder
- ¾ cup water
- 1 tomato, chopped

**Directions:**
Place all the ingredients in the instant pot bowl. Close the lid and set the "Manual" mode (High Pressure). Cook the meal for 50 minutes. Then make natural pressure release. Serve the meal immediately!

**Nutrition value/serving:** calories 370, fat 13.4, fiber 2.3, carbs 7.4, protein 52.8

## Basil Beef Ribs

*Prep time: 10 minutes | Cooking time: 25 minutes | Servings: 2*

**Ingredients:**
- 1 teaspoon dried basil
- 10 oz beef ribs
- ¾ cup water
- 1 teaspoon butter
- 1 teaspoon ground black pepper
- ½ teaspoon salt
- 1 onion, diced
- ¼ teaspoon dried rosemary

**Directions:**
Rub the beef ribs with the ground black pepper. Salt, and dried rosemary. Place the beef ribs in the instant pot bowl. Add diced onion, butter, and water. Close the lid and set "Meat" mode. Cook the ribs for 20 minutes – to get the tender taste. Chill the meat for 5 minutes and serve!

**Nutrition value/serving:** calories 305, fat 10.9, fiber 1.5, carbs 5.9, protein 43.8

# Buffalo Chicken Soup

*Prep time: 7 minutes | Cooking time: 10 minutes | Servings: 2*

**Ingredients:**

- 6 oz chicken, cooked
- 2 oz Parmesan, shredded
- 4 tablespoons full-fat cream
- ¼ teaspoon ground black pepper
- ¾ teaspoon salt
- 2 tablespoons Red Hot sauce
- 1 oz celery stalk, chopped
- 1 cup water

**Directions:**

Place the chopped celery stalk, water, salt, ground black pepper, full-fat cream, and cheese in the instant pot. Stir it gently. Lock the instant pot lid and seal it. Set the "Manual" mode (High pressure) and turn on the timer for 7 minutes. Shred the cooked chicken and combine it together with Red Hot Sauce. When the soup is cooked make quick pressure release and ladle the soup on the bowls. Add shredded chicken and serve!

**Nutrition value/serving:** calories 263, fat 12.2, fiber 0.3, carbs 3.1, protein 34.9

# Greek-Style Chicken Thighs

*Prep time: 7 minutes | Cooking time: 15 minutes | Servings: 2*

**Ingredients:**

- 4 lemon slices
- 2 chicken thighs
- 1 tablespoon Greek seasoning
- ½ white onion, diced
- 1 teaspoon butter
- ½ cup water

**Directions:**

Rub the chicken thighs with Greek seasoning and diced onion. Then spread the chicken with butter. Pour water in the instant pot and place the trivet. Place the chicken on the foil and top with the lemon slices. Wrap the chicken in the foil and transfer on the trivet. Set the "Saute" mode and lock the instant pot lid. Seal it. Cook the meal for 10 minutes. Then make quick pressure release for 5 minutes. Discard the foil from the chicken thighs and serve!

**Nutrition value/serving:** calories 320, fat 13, fiber 1, carbs 6.1, protein 43

## Butter Prawns

*Prep time: 5 minutes | Cooking time: 6 minutes | Servings: 2*

**Ingredients:**
- 1 teaspoon smoked paprika
- 1 teaspoon ground paprika
- 12 oz prawns
- 1 teaspoon butter
- ½ cup cream
- ½ teaspoon chili flakes

**Directions:**
Set the "Saute" mode and toss the butter in the instant pot bowl. Melt it. Then add prawns and sprinkle them with the ground paprika, smoked paprika, and chili flakes. Stir well and cook for 3 minutes. After this, add cream and lock the instant pot lid. Cook the meal for 3 minutes (QR). Serve the prawns with gravy.

**Nutrition value/serving:** calories 261, fat 8.3, fiber 0.4, carbs 5.1, protein 39.4

## Bacon Chowder

*Prep time: 5 minutes | Cooking time: 8 minutes | Servings: 2*

**Ingredients:**
- 1 cup full-fat cream
- 1 tablespoon cream cheese
- 4 oz bacon, chopped, fried
- 1 oz celery stalk
- ¼ teaspoon salt
- 1 teaspoon turmeric

**Directions:**
Pour the full-fat cream in the instant pot bowl. Chop the celery stalk and add it in the instant pot bowl too. After this, add salt, turmeric, and cream cheese. Lock the instant pot lid and seal it. Press the "Manual" mode (High pressure) and set the timer for 3 minutes. Then make naturally pressure release for 5 minutes. Ladle the chowder in the bowls and add fried bacon.

**Nutrition value/serving:** calories 488, fat 39.5, fiber 0.5, carbs 7.3, protein 25.2

## Chicken Stew with Mushrooms

*Prep time: 10 minutes | Cooking time: 30 minutes | Servings: 2*

**Ingredients:**

- 10 oz chicken breast, skinless, boneless
- 4 oz mushrooms
- ¼ teaspoon salt
- ½ teaspoon white pepper
- ¾ teaspoon garlic powder
- ½ teaspoon butter
- ¾ cup water
- 1 tablespoon full-fat cream

**Directions:**

Chop the chicken breast roughly and place in the instant pot bowl. Add salt, white pepper, garlic powder, and water. Set "Saute" mode and start to cook the poultry. Meanwhile, slice the mushrooms. Add mushrooms in the instant pot bowl. Add full-fat cream and stir it. Close the lid and seal it. Set the timer on 25 minutes.

**Nutrition value/serving:** calories 197, fat 5.6, fiber 0.8, carbs 3.3, protein 32.3

## Mongolian Beef

*Prep time: 8 minutes | Cooking time: 13 minutes | Servings: 2*

**Ingredients:**

- 14 oz beef flank steak
- 1 tablespoon almond flour
- ½ onion, chopped
- ½ teaspoon minced ginger
- ½ teaspoon minced garlic
- ½ teaspoon chili flakes
- 1 tablespoon butter
- ¾ cup water

**Directions:**

Cut the flank steak into the strips. Then toss the beef strips in the almond flour and shake well. Toss the butter in the instant pot bowl and set the "saute" mode. When the butter is melted – add the beef flank steak strips and cook them for 3 minutes. Stir them time to time. Meanwhile, mix up together the minced garlic, minced ginger, chili flakes, and butter. Add chopped onion. Pour the liquid over the meat and lock the instant pot lid. Press the "Manual" mode (High pressure) and set the timer for 10 minutes. Make a quick pressure release and serve the meat!

**Nutrition value/serving:** calories 470, fat 24.1, fiber 1.1, carbs 3.9, protein 56.4

## Tuna Casserole

*Prep time: 7 minutes | Cooking time: 5 minutes | Servings: 2*

**Ingredients:**
- ½ green pepper
- 1 teaspoon chili flakes
- 10 oz tuna
- 1 tablespoon cream cheese
- ½ teaspoon salt
- 5 oz Parmesan, shredded
- 1 teaspoon butter

**Directions:**
Cut the green peppers into the strips. Take the springform pan and grease it with the butter. Make the layer of tuna in the springform pan. After this, put the layer of the shredded cheese, Add green pepper. Sprinkle the casserole with the salt and chili flakes. Repeat the same steps with the remaining ingredients. Top the casserole with the cream cheese. Pour 1 cup of water in the instant pot bowl and place the trivet. Put the casserole on the trivet and wrap with the foil. Lock the instant pot lid and seal it. Set "Manual" mode (High pressure) for 5 minutes. Make a quick pressure release. Chill the casserole little and serve!

**Nutrition value/serving:** calories 532, fat 30.3, fiber 0.5, carbs 4.1, protein 61.1


## Stuffed Mushrooms with Cheese

*Prep time: 5 minutes | Cooking time: 5 minutes | Servings: 2*

**Ingredients:**
- 4 white mushrooms hats
- 1 teaspoon butter
- 1 tablespoon fresh dill, chopped
- 1/3 teaspoon salt
- ¾ teaspoon chili pepper
- 3 oz Cheddar cheese, shredded

**Directions:**
Peel the mushroom hats. Churn together the butter, fresh dill, salt, and chili pepper. Dill the mushroom hats with the butter mixture. Then top the mushrooms with the shredded cheese. Wrap every mushroom hat in the foil. Pour ½ cup of water in the instant pot bowl and place the trivet. Put the mushrooms on the trivet and lock the instant pot lid. Seal it. Set the "Manual" mode (High pressure) and cook mushrooms for 5 minutes. Then make quick pressure release. Discard the mushrooms from the foil and serve them hot!

**Nutrition value/serving:** calories 201, fat 16.2, fiber 0.7, carbs 2.8, protein 12.1

## Zucchini Salad

*Prep time: 5 minutes | Cooking time: 6 minutes | Servings: 2*

**Ingredients:**
- 1 zucchini, chopped
- 5 oz chicken breast, chopped
- 1 tablespoon butter
- 1 tablespoon lemon juice
- ½ teaspoon chili flakes
- 1 tablespoon fresh dill, chopped
- ½ cucumber
- ¾ cup water

**Directions:**

Toss the butter in the instant pot and preheat it on "Saute" mode. Add chopped chicken breast. Sprinkle it with the chili flakes and cook for 4 minutes. Then add chopped zucchini and water; close the lid. Seal the lid and set the "Manual" mode; press timer for 3 minutes (High Pressure). Make the quick pressure release then. Chop the cucumber and place in the salad bowl. Add fresh dill and lemon juice. After this, add chicken breast and zucchini (don't use the remaining gravy). Stir the salad directly before serving.

**Nutrition value/serving:** calories 165, fat 7.9, fiber 1.7, carbs 7.1, protein 17.1

## Fabulous Seabass Steak

*Prep time: 5 minutes | Cooking time: 3 minutes | Servings: 2*

**Ingredients:**
- 14 oz seabass steak
- ½ teaspoon dried thyme
- ¾ teaspoon salt
- ¾ teaspoon dried rosemary
- ¾ cup coconut milk
- ½ teaspoon minced garlic
- ½ teaspoon smoked paprika

**Directions:**

Mix up together the dried thyme, salt, dried rosemary, minced garlic, and smoked paprika. Rub the seabass steak with the spice mixture. Place the seabass in the instant pot bowl. Add coconut milk and lock the instant pot lid. Set the "Manual" mode for 3 minutes. Make the quick-release pressure then. Serve the fish immediately!

**Nutrition value/serving:** calories 618, fat 46, fiber 4, carbs 6.2, protein 47.3

# Fish Cakes

*Prep time: 8 minutes | **Cooking time:** 5 minutes | **Servings:** 2*

**Ingredients:**
- 1 tablespoon butter
- 15 oz cod
- ¼ teaspoon minced garlic
- ½ teaspoon dried dill
- ¼ onion, diced

**Directions:**

Chop the cod into the tiny pieces and combine together with the minced garlic, dried dill, and diced onion. Toss the butter in the instant pot bowl and preheat it on "Saute" mode. Meanwhile, make the medium fish cakes from the cod mixture. Place the fish cakes in the melted butter and cook for 1 minute from each side. After this, lock the lid and cook the fish cakes for 3 minutes.

**Nutrition value/serving:** calories 281, fat 7.6, fiber 0.3, carbs 1.5, protein 48.8

# Salmon Quiche

*Prep time: 7 minutes | **Cooking time:** 10 minutes | **Servings:** 2*

**Ingredients:**
- 2 eggs, beaten
- 12 oz salmon fillet
- 1 tablespoon cream cheese
- ¾ teaspoon dried rosemary
- 1 teaspoon fresh dill, chopped
- ½ teaspoon ground white pepper
- ¼ teaspoon salt
- 1 teaspoon butter

**Directions:**

Chop the salmon into the ½ inch size pieces. Whisk the beaten eggs until homogenous. Add the cream cheese, dried rosemary, dill, white pepper, and salt. Grease the springform with the butter and place the layer of the salmon. Pour the egg mixture over the salmon and close the lid. Set the "Manual" mode (High pressure) and cook for 5 minutes. Then make natural-release pressure for 5 minutes. Cut the quiche into the serving and enjoy!

**Nutrition value/serving:** calories 326, fat 18.6, fiber 0.4, carbs 1.4, protein 39.1

## Asian Meatballs

*Prep time: 10 minutes | Cooking time: 7 minutes | Servings: 2*

**Ingredients:**

- 1 white onion, chopped
- 11 oz ground pork
- 1 teaspoon lemon juice
- ¼ teaspoon fish sauce
- ½ teaspoon ground black pepper
- ¼ teaspoon chili flakes
- 1 tablespoon butter
- 3 tablespoons water
- ¼ teaspoon fresh ginger, minced

**Directions:**

Combine together the ground pork and chopped onion. Add lemon juice, fish sauce, ground black pepper, and chili flakes. After this, add fresh ginger and mix up the mixture very well. Toss the butter in the instant pot bowl and melt it. Meanwhile, make the small meatballs from the meat mixture. Place the meatballs in the instant pot and cook for 2 minutes from each side. After this, add water and lock the lid. Set the "Manual" mode for 3 minutes (High pressure). When the time is over – make the quick-release pressure.

**Nutrition value/serving:** calories 299, fat 11.3, fiber 1.4, carbs 5.7, protein 41.6

## Garam Masala

*Prep time: 5 minutes | Cooking time: 4 minutes | Servings: 2*

**Ingredients:**

- ¼ teaspoon ground cumin
- ½ teaspoon turmeric
- 1 teaspoon ground paprika
- ¾ teaspoon chili flakes
- ½ teaspoon cardamom
- ¾ teaspoon ground nutmeg
- ½ teaspoon ground coriander
- ½ cup coconut milk
- 14 oz chicken breast, skinless, boneless
- 1 green pepper, chopped
- 1 tablespoon butter

**Directions:**

Blend together the ground cumin, turmeric, ground paprika, chili flakes, cardamom, ground nutmeg, coriander, coconut milk, green pepper, and butter. When the mixture is smooth – pour it in the instant pot bowl. Chop the chicken breast roughly and transfer it in the spice mixture. Stir gently with the help of the spatula. Lock the lid and seal it. Set the "Manual" mode for 4 minutes (High pressure). After this, make quick-release pressure.

**Nutrition value/serving:** calories 439, fat 25.7, fiber 3.2, carbs 7.9, protein 44.4

## Pulled Pork

*Prep time: 7 minutes | Cooking time: 40 minutes | Servings: 2*

**Ingredients:**

- 1-pound pork roast, chopped
- ½ teaspoon ground cumin
- ½ teaspoon turmeric
- ½ teaspoon ground coriander
- ½ teaspoon ground black pepper
- 1 teaspoon smoked paprika
- ½ teaspoon white pepper
- 1 cup beef broth
- 1 tablespoon butter
- 1 teaspoon onion powder

**Directions:**

Mix up together all the spices. Then combine together the spices and chopped pork roast. Place the meat in the instant pot bowl. Add butter and beef broth. Close the instant pot lid and seal it. Set the manual mode and put the timer on 30 minutes (High pressure). When the time is over – make the natural-release pressure. Transfer the cooked meat in the bowl and shred it. Add the small amount of the remaining gravy and serve!

**Nutrition value/serving:** calories 556, fat 28.2, fiber 1.1, carbs 3.8, protein 67.7

## Lamb Stew

*Prep time: 5 minutes | Cooking time: 50 minutes | Servings: 2*

**Ingredients:**

- ½ cup coconut milk
- 1 teaspoon butter
- ½ teaspoon dried rosemary
- ¼ teaspoon salt
- ½ teaspoon ground coriander
- ½ teaspoon ground cumin
- 13 oz lamb shoulder, chopped
- 1 garlic clove, chopped
- 4 oz mushrooms
- ¾ cup water

**Directions:**

Slice the mushrooms and place them in the instant pot bowl. Add chopped garlic, water, lamb shoulder, ground cumin, ground coriander, salt, dried rosemary, and coconut milk. After this, add butter and lock the instant pot lid. Seal it and set "Manual" mode for 45 minutes. When the time is over – make natural-release pressure for 5 minutes. Serve the stew immediately!

**Nutrition value/serving:** calories 515, fat 30.1, fiber 2.1, carbs 6.1, protein 55.1

# Rosemary Chicken Wings

*Prep time:* 7 *minutes* | *Cooking time:* 10 *minutes* | *Servings:* 2

## Ingredients:

- 1 teaspoon dried rosemary
- 1 teaspoon cream cheese
- ½ green pepper
- ½ teaspoon turmeric
- ½ teaspoon salt
- ½ teaspoon ground black pepper
- 14 oz chicken wings
- ¾ cup water
- 1 teaspoon butter

## Directions:

Rub the chicken wings with the dried rosemary, turmeric, salt, and ground black pepper. Blend the green pepper until you get a puree. Rub the chicken wings in the green pepper puree. Then toss the butter in the instant pot bowl and preheat it on the "Saute" mode. Add the chicken wings and cook them for 3 minutes from each side or until light brown. Then add cream cheese and water. Lock the instant pot lid and seal it. Set the "Manual" mode and put the timer for 4 minutes (High Pressure). When the time is over – make the quick-release pressure. Let the cooked chicken wings chill for 1-2 minutes and serve them!

**Nutrition value/serving:** calories 411, fat 17.4, fiber 1, carbs 2.5, protein 58

# Side Dishes

## Tender Mashed Cauliflower
*Prep time: 8 minutes | Cooking time: 5 minutes | Servings: 2*

**Ingredients:**
- ½ cup coconut milk
- 1 teaspoon butter
- ½ teaspoon salt
- ¼ teaspoon turmeric
- 10 oz cauliflower, chopped

**Directions:**
Place the chopped cauliflower in the instant pot. Add salt, turmeric, butter, and coconut milk. Set the "Manual" mode (High pressure) on the instant pot. Set the timer for 5 minutes. When the time is over – use the quick pressure release method. Transfer the cauliflower (without liquid) in the blender. Blend it until smooth. After this, transfer the cauliflower mash in the bowl. Start to add a small amount of the remaining liquid from the instant pot. Stir the cauliflower mash well and add more liquid if you think that the meal is not soft enough. Serve the cauliflower mash warm!

**Nutrition value/serving:** calories 191, fat 16.4, fiber 4.9, carbs 11, protein 4.2

## Spicy Courgette Zoodles
*Prep time: 10 minutes | Cooking time: 10 minutes | Servings: 2*

**Ingredients:**
- 1 cup water
- 14 oz courgette
- 1 tablespoon butter
- ½ teaspoon salt

**Directions:**
Cut the courgette into halves. Pour 1 cup of water in the instant pot and place the trivet. Sprinkle the vegetable with the salt and add butter. Transfer the courgette on the trivet and close the lid. Set the "Steam" mode + High Pressure. Cook the vegetable for 10 minutes. After this, make quick pressure release. Transfer the courgette on the plate and fluff out the zoodles with the help of the fork. Throw away the courgette skin. Serve the side dish immediately!

**Nutrition value/serving:** calories 83, fat 6.1, fiber 2.2, carbs 6.7, protein 2.5

## Zucchini Zoodles with Chilli Pepper
*Prep time: 7 minutes | Cooking time: 3 minutes | Servings: 2*

**Ingredients:**
- 1 teaspoon chili pepper
- 2 zucchini
- ½ cup chicken stock
- 1 teaspoon butter
- ½ teaspoon salt

**Directions:**
Wash the zucchini well. Make the noodles from the zucchini with the help of the spiralizer. Sprinkle zucchini noodles with the salt and chili pepper. Place the chicken stock and butter in the instant pot bowl and preheat the liquid on "Saute" mode. Add the spiralized zucchini and cook on "Manual" mode; set timer on Zero –QR. Chill the zoodles little and serve!

**Nutrition value/serving:** calories 52, fat 2.4, fiber 2.3, carbs 7, protein 2.6


## White Mushrooms Saute
*Prep time: 8 minutes | Cooking time: 25 minutes | Servings: 2*

**Ingredients:**
- 2 teaspoons butter
- 7 oz white mushrooms, sliced
- 3 tablespoon coconut milk
- ½ teaspoon white pepper
- ¼ teaspoon turmeric

**Directions:**
Melt the butter in the instant pot bowl on "Saute" mode. Add coconut milk, white pepper, turmeric, and stir well. Preheat the liquid until it starts to boil. Add sliced mushrooms and stir well with the help of the wooden spatula. After this, close the lid and cook the saute on "Saute" mode for 20 minutes. Reduce the time of cooking if you want the solid texture of the mushrooms. Serve the saute with gravy.

**Nutrition value/serving:** calories 111, fat 9.2, fiber 1.9, carbs 5.2, protein 4.1

# Celery Ragout

*Prep time: 6 minutes | Cooking time: 15 minutes | Servings: 2*

**Ingredients:**
- 7 oz celery stalk, chopped
- 1 cup spinach, chopped
- 1 garlic clove, chopped
- ½ teaspoon ground coriander
- ½ teaspoon salt
- ¾ teaspoon ground cinnamon
- ¾ cup almond milk
- ½ teaspoon chili pepper

**Directions:**
Chop the celery stalk and spinach roughly and sprinkle the vegetables with the ground coriander, salt, ground cinnamon, and chili pepper. Add garlic clove and transfer the ingredients in the instant pot. Add almond milk and close the lid. Cook the ragout on "Saute" mode for 15 minutes to get the soft vegetable texture. Serve the meal warm.

**Nutrition value/serving:** calories 231, fat 21.7, fiber 4.4, carbs 9.8, protein 3.3

# Sauteed Spinach

*Prep time: 5 minutes | Cooking time: 10 minutes | Servings: 2*

**Ingredients:**
- 2 cups spinach
- 1 oz pecans, crushed
- ½ cup chicken stock
- 1 teaspoon cream cheese
- ½ teaspoon salt
- ½ teaspoon ground black pepper

**Directions:**
Pour the chicken stock in the instant pot bowl. Add cream cheese, salt, ground black pepper, and crushed pecans. Wash the spinach well and chop it very roughly. Place the spinach in the chicken stock and close the lid. Cook the meal on "Saute" mode for 10 minutes (QR). Discard the spinach from the chicken stock gravy and transfer on the plates.

**Nutrition value/serving:** calories 115, fat 1, fiber 2.3, carbs 3.7, protein 2.7

# Fragrant Asparagus

*Prep time: 6 minutes | Cooking time: 4 minutes | Servings: 2*

## Ingredients:

- 9 oz asparagus
- ¼ teaspoon ground black pepper
- 1 teaspoon butter
- 1 teaspoon chili flakes
- ¾ teaspoon minced garlic
- 2 oz Parmesan, shredded

## Directions:

Grease the springform pan with butter. Place the asparagus in the springform pan. Sprinkle the vegetables with the chili flakes, minced garlic, and ground black pepper. Close the lid and set the "Manual" mode (High pressure) for 4 minutes. When the asparagus is cooked – make quick pressure release. Transfer the asparagus on the serving plates immediately and sprinkle with the shredded cheese.

**Nutrition value/serving:** calories 136, fat 8.2, fiber 2.8, carbs 6.5, protein 12.1

# Tender Cauliflower Florets

*Prep time: 5 minutes | Cooking time: 1 minute | Servings: 2*

## Ingredients:

- ¼ teaspoon fresh ginger, minced
- ½ teaspoon minced garlic
- 1 teaspoon butter
- ½ teaspoon salt
- ¾ teaspoon chili flakes
- 1 teaspoon fresh dill, chopped
- 10 oz cauliflower

## Directions:

Cut the cauliflower into the florets and sprinkle with the chili flakes, fresh dill, salt, and minced garlic. Add butter and minced ginger. Mix up the vegetables. Place the vegetables into the steamer basket and put in the instant pot. Close the lid and set "Manual" mode (High pressure); cook the meal for 1 minute. Then make quick pressure release.

**Nutrition value/serving:** calories 56, fat 2.1, fiber 3.7, carbs 8.2, protein 3

## Butter Green Beans

*Prep time: 5 minutes | **Cooking time:** 3 minutes | **Servings:** 2*

**Ingredients:**
- 2 teaspoons butter
- 11 oz green beans
- 4 tablespoons full-fat cream
- ¾ cup fresh parsley, chopped

**Directions:**

Churn together the butter, full-fat cream, and parsley. Chop the green beans roughly. Place the green beans in the steamer basket and close the instant pot. Set the "Manual" mode (High pressure) and put time for 2 minutes. When the time is over – make quick pressure release. Transfer the hot green beans on the plate and add churned butter mixture.

**Nutrition value/serving:** calories 117, fat 6.8, fiber 5.6, carbs 13, protein 3.7

## Curry Cabbage

*Prep time: 7 minutes | **Cooking time:** 15 minutes | **Servings:** 2*

**Ingredients:**
- 1 tablespoon curry
- 10 oz white cabbage, shredded
- 1 teaspoon butter
- 3 tablespoons cream cheese
- ½ teaspoon salt

**Directions:**

Place the cabbage in the big mixing bowl. Sprinkle the cabbage with the curry and salt. Stir well with the help of the fingertips. Melt the butter on "Saute" mode in the instant pot. Add cream cheese and stir until homogenous. Then add all the shredded cabbage and stir gently. Transfer the cabbage mixture in the cake pan. Pour ½ cup of water in the instant pot. Insert the trivet. Transfer the cake pan on the trivet and lock the instant pot lid. Set the "steam" mode and cook the cabbage for 10 minutes. Transfer the cooked meal on the serving plates.

**Nutrition value/serving:** calories 115, fat 7.7, fiber 4.6, carbs 10.5, protein 3.4

## Eggplants Stew

*Prep time: 10 minutes | Cooking time: 25 minutes | Servings: 2*

**Ingredients:**

- 8 oz eggplant
- ½ white onion, chopped
- 1 tablespoon butter
- ½ teaspoon salt
- ½ tomato, chopped
- ½ teaspoon ground black pepper
- 2 oz Parmesan, shredded

**Directions:**

Wash the eggplant carefully and cut it into the medium cubes. Sprinkle the eggplant with the salt and ground black pepper. Stir it carefully with the help of fingertips. Leave the eggplants for 5 minutes. Meanwhile, toss the butter in the instant pot; turn on "Saute" mode and melt the butter. Add chopped onion and eggplant. After this, add tomato and close the lid. Saute the stew for 20 minutes. Transfer the cooked meal on the plates and sprinkle with the cheese.

**Nutrition value/serving:** calories 186, fat 12.1, fiber 4.9, carbs 11.2, protein 10.8

## Tender Kale

*Prep time: 5 minutes | Cooking time: 5 minutes | Servings: 2*

**Ingredients:**

- 10 oz kale, Italian dark-leaf
- 3 tablespoons butter
- ½ teaspoon chili powder
- ¾ teaspoon garlic powder

**Directions:**

Set the "Saute" mode at the instant pot. Place butter, garlic powder, and chili powder in the instant pot bowl and cook it until butter is melted. Then chop the kale roughly and add in the instant pot too. Mix up the mixture with the help of the wooden spatula and lock the lid. Cook the kale on "Manual" mode for 3 minutes (High pressure – QR).

**Nutrition value/serving:** calories 195, fat 17.9, fiber 2.9, carbs 8.5, protein 2.9

# Keto Bok Choy

*Prep time: 5 minutes | **Cooking time:** 7 minutes | **Servings:** 2*

**Ingredients:**
- 2 cups bok choy, chopped
- 1 teaspoon butter
- ½ tablespoon cream cheese
- ¼ teaspoon minced ginger
- ¾ teaspoon salt

**Directions:**

Preheat the instant pot on the "Saute" mode. Add butter and minced garlic. Saute the ingredients for 1 minute. After this, add salt, cream cheese, and chopped bok choy. Stir the meal well and saute for 3 minutes. Then lock the instant pot lid and set "Manual" mode. Set timer for 3 minutes (High pressure) – QR. Serve the bok choy warm!

**Nutrition value/serving:** calories 35, fat 2.9, fiber 0.7, carbs 1.8, protein 1.3

# Kale-Feta Saute

*Prep time: 5 minutes | **Cooking time:** 6 minutes | **Servings:** 2*

**Ingredients:**
- 1 cup Kale, Italian dark-leaf
- 3 oz tofu, chopped
- 1 teaspoon butter
- ½ teaspoon flax meal
- ½ teaspoon salt
- ¾ teaspoon ground nutmeg
- 1 oz Feta
- 1/3 cup water

**Directions:**

Wash and chop the kale roughly. Toss butter in the instant pot bowl and melt it on "Saute" mode. Add the chopped kale. Sprinkle the kale leaves with the salt and ground nutmeg. Add water and flax meal. Stir the kale well with the help of a spatula. Lock the instant pot lid and seal it. Set the "Manual" mode (High pressure) for 4 minutes. When the meal is cooked – make the quick-release pressure. Crumble Feta cheese. Transfer the cooked kale on the serving plates and sprinkle with the crumbled cheese.

**Nutrition value/serving:** calories 107, fat 7.2, fiber 1.2, carbs 5.4, protein 6.7

# Hash Brown

*Prep time: 6 minutes | Cooking time: 9 minutes | Servings: 2*

## Ingredients:

- 8 oz cauliflower, shredded
- 1 egg, beaten
- ½ teaspoon cayenne pepper
- 2 oz Parmesan cheese, shredded
- ¼ teaspoon chili flakes
- 1 tablespoon butter

## Directions:

Combine together the shredded cauliflower and beaten egg. Stir the mixture until homogenous. Add cayenne pepper, shredded cheese, chili flakes, and butter. Stir the mixture with the help of a spatula. After this, transfer the mixture in the non-sticky springform pan or cake mold. Place the pan in the instant pot and cover with the foil. Lock the instant pot lid and seal it. Set the "Manual" mode – High Pressure. Cook hash brown for 4 minutes. Then make naturally pressure release for 5 minutes.

**Nutrition value/serving:** calories 203, fat 14.2, fiber 3, carbs 7.5, protein 14.2

# Cabbage Petals

*Prep time: 5 minutes | Cooking time: 4 minutes | Servings: 2*

## Ingredients:

- 7 oz white cabbage
- 1 oz bacon, fried, chopped
- ½ teaspoon onion powder
- ¼ teaspoon salt
- ¾ teaspoon chili flakes
- 1 teaspoon butter
- 5 tablespoons coconut milk
- 1 teaspoon mustard

## Directions:

Cut the cabbage into the petals and sprinkle with salt, chili flakes, and onion powder. Place the cabbage into the instant pot. Add butter and coconut milk. If there is not enough liquid – add water. Close the lid and set "Manual" mode (High Pressure) for 4 minutes. Then make quick pressure release. Transfer the cooked cabbage petals in the bowl and add mustard and fried bacon. Stir the meal.

**Nutrition value/serving:** calories 215, fat 17.4, fiber 3.6, carbs 9.1, protein 7.9

# Coconut Milk Broccoli

*Prep time: 6 minutes* | *Cooking time: 18 minutes* | *Servings: 2*

**Ingredients:**

- 1 teaspoon salt
- 8 oz broccoli
- ¾ cup coconut milk
- ¼ cup water
- ½ teaspoon butter
- 1 teaspoon cayenne pepper

**Directions:**

Cut the broccoli into the medium pieces and place in the instant pot. Add butter and start to saute it for 3 minutes on "Saute" mode. Then add cayenne pepper, salt, and coconut milk. Stir gently and close the lead. Cook the meal on "Saute mode" for 15 minutes. Remove the cooked broccoli from the instant pot immediately (to prevent the overcooking). Serve the broccoli with the small amount of gravy.

**Nutrition value/serving:** calories 223, fat 22.6, fiber 2.6, carbs 6.5, protein 2.6

# Stuffed Celery Stalks with Goat Cheese

*Prep time: 6 minutes* | *Cooking time: 4 minutes* | *Servings: 2*

**Ingredients:**

- 7 oz celery stalks
- 4 oz goat cheese
- 1 garlic clove, minced
- ¼ teaspoon paprika
- 1 oz Parmesan, grated

**Directions:**

Cut the celery stalks on the medium boats. After this, mix up together the grated cheese, paprika, minced garlic, and goat cheese. Churn the mixture. Fill the celery boats with the cheese mixture and place on the instant pot rack. Pour 1 cup of water in the instant pot and transfer the rack with the celery stalks. Close the lid and cook on the "Steam" mode for 4 minutes.

**Nutrition value/serving:** calories 321, fat 23.4, fiber 1.7, carbs 5.3, protein 22.7

# Roasted Fennel Salad

*Prep time: 5 minutes | **Cooking time:** 5 minutes | **Servings:** 2*

## Ingredients:
- 1 fennel bulb, chopped
- ¾ cup fresh parsley, chopped
- 1 tablespoon butter
- 1 teaspoon apple cider vinegar
- ¼ teaspoon ground black pepper
- 1 oz tofu, chopped
- ½ oz olives
- 2 tablespoons coconut milk

## Directions:
Set the "Saute" mode at the instant pot and toss the butter inside. Add chopped fennel, apple cider vinegar, and ground black pepper. Saute the vegetable for 4 minutes or until soft. Add coconut milk and cook it for 1 minute more. Meanwhile, chop the parsley and slice the olives. Transfer the ingredients in the salad bowl. Add cook fennel and a small amount of fennel gravy (for seasoning). Mix it up directly before serving.

**Nutrition value/serving:** calories 149, fat 11.1, fiber 5.1, carbs 11.7, protein 3.8

# Cauliflower Rice

*Prep time: 5 minutes | **Cooking time:** 5 minutes | **Servings:** 2*

## Ingredients:
- ¾ cup coconut milk
- 8 oz cauliflower, shredded
- 1 teaspoon butter
- ½ teaspoon salt

## Directions:
Put the butter in the instant pot and preheat it on "Saute" mode. Add shredded cauliflower and salt. Stir the mixture and cook for 1 minute more. After this, add coconut milk, mix up the ingredients and lock the instant pot. Set the "Manual" mode (High pressure) and cook the side dish for 3 minutes. After this, make quick pressure release (follow the directions of your instant pot). Transfer the cooked cauliflower rice in the serving plates.

**Nutrition value/serving:** calories 252, fat 23.5, fiber 4.8, carbs 11, protein 4.3

# Asian Noodles

*Prep time: 5 minutes | **Cooking time:** 1 minute | **Servings:** 2*

**Ingredients:**
- 7 oz Konjac Noodles
- 1 teaspoon butter, melted
- ½ teaspoon apple cider vinegar

**Directions:**
Rinse Konjac Noodles carefully under the warm water. Place the butter in the instant pot bowl and add noodles. Add apple cider vinegar. Close the lid and set the "Manual" mode (High pressure) for 1 minute. When the time is over – use the quick pressure release method. Serve the noodles hot!

**Nutrition value/serving:** calories 26, fat 11.9, fiber 3, carbs 3.5, protein 0

# Broccoli Mash

*Prep time: 5 minutes | **Cooking time:** 7 minutes | **Servings:** 2*

**Ingredients:**
- 6 oz broccoli
- ½ teaspoon salt
- 1 teaspoon butter

**Directions:**
Cut the broccoli into the florets and place in the steamer basket. Pour 1 cup of water in the instant pot bowl and add steamer basket. Close the lid and cook in "Steam" mode for 7 minutes. After this, mix up together the cooked broccoli, salt, and butter. Blend the mixture well with the help of the hand blender. When you get the smooth and fluffy texture – the mash is cooked.

**Nutrition value/serving:** calories 46, fat 2.2, fiber 2.2, carbs 5.7, protein 2.4

## Thyme Salmon Salad

*Prep time: 5 minutes | Cooking time: 4 minutes | Servings: 2*

**Ingredients:**

- 1 teaspoon ground thyme
- ½ teaspoon salt
- 6 oz salmon

- 2 cups lettuce
- 1 teaspoon almond milk
- ½ teaspoon mustard

**Directions:**

Sprinkle the salmon with salt and wrap in foil. Place the salmon on the trivet and transfer in the instant pot bowl. Add ½ cup of water in the instant bowl and close the lid. Cook the salmon on "Manual" mode (High Pressure) for 4 minutes (QR). Meanwhile, tear the lettuce and toss it in the salad bowl. Whisk together the almond milk, mustard, and ground thyme. When the salmon is cooked – discard it from the foil and chop roughly. Place the salmon over the lettuce and sprinkle with the almond milk seasoning.

**Nutrition value/serving:** calories 131, fat 6.2, fiber 0.7, carbs 2.4, protein 17.1

## Egg Salad

*Prep time: 5 minutes | Cooking time: 4 minutes | Servings: 2*

**Ingredients:**

- 1 cup lettuce
- 1 tomato, chopped
- 2 eggs

- 1 teaspoon mustard
- ¼ teaspoon onion powder
- 2 tablespoons coconut milk

**Directions:**

Pour 1 cup of water in the instant pot and add eggs. Close the lid and cook the eggs on the "Manual" mode for 5 minutes (high pressure – quick pressure release). Meanwhile, tear the lettuce and place in the bowl. Add chopped tomato. Mix up together the mustard, onion powder, and coconut milk. Add the mustard sauce in the lettuce salad. When the eggs are cooked – chill them in the cold water and pell. Cut each egg into 4 parts and add in the salad.

**Nutrition value/serving:** calories 116, fat 8.5, fiber 1.1, carbs 4, protein 6.7

# Zucchini Boats with Cheese

*Prep time: 5 minutes | **Cooking time:** 3 minutes | Servings: 2*

**Ingredients:**

- 1 zucchini
- 3 oz Parmesan
- 1 tablespoon fresh dill, chopped
- 2 teaspoon butter, softened
- 1 teaspoon chili flakes
- 2 tablespoon water

**Directions:**

Cut the zucchini into 2 parts and remove the pulp with the help of the spoon. Grate Parmesan and combine it together with the softened butter, chili flakes, water, and fresh dill. Stir well. Fill the zucchini boats with the cheese mixture and then wrap the vegetables in the foil. Each zucchini boat wrap in the separated foil. Place the zucchini into the instant pot and close the lid. Seal the lid. Set the "Manual" mode (High Pressure) and cook the "boats" for 4 minutes. After this, use the quick pressure method. Let the zucchini boats chill for 3-4 minutes. Then discard the foil and serve the side dish.

**Nutrition value/serving:** calories 190, fat 13.2, fiber 1.3, carbs 5.7, protein 15.2

# Main Dishes

## Chili Verde

*Prep time: 10 minutes | Cooking time: 40 minutes | Servings: 2*

**Ingredients:**

- 12 oz pork shoulder
- ½ cup salsa verde
- 1 tablespoon butter
- 

- ¼ cup chicken stock
- ¾ teaspoon white pepper
- ½ teaspoon salt

**Directions:**

Chop the pork shoulder and sprinkle the meat with the white pepper and salt. Toss the butter in the instant pot and saute it for 1 minute or until it is melted. After this, add pork shoulder and saute it for 10 minutes. After this, add chicken stock and salsa verde. Lock the instant pot lid and seal it. Set the "Bean/Chili" mode and set the timer on 30 minutes (High Pressure). When the time is over – make a natural pressure release.

**Nutrition value/serving:** calories 566, fat 42.4, fiber 0.5, carbs 3.2, protein 40.6

## Chicken Tikka Masala

*Prep time: 10 minutes | Cooking time: 25 minutes | Servings: 2*

**Ingredients:**

- 14 oz chicken breast
- ½ white onion, diced
- ½ teaspoon ground cardamom
- ¼ teaspoon ground coriander
- ¾ teaspoon minced ginger

- ½ cup full-fat cream
- ½ teaspoon salt
- ¼ teaspoon ground black pepper
- ¾ teaspoon nutmeg
- 1 teaspoon butter

**Directions:**

Mix up together the diced onion, ground cardamom, ground coriander, minced garlic, minced ginger, ground black pepper, and nutmeg. Then chop the chicken breast roughly. Stir the spice mixture in the full-fat cream and whisk until homogenous. Place the butter and chicken in the instant pot bowl. Add full-fat cream and lock the instant pot lid. Set the "Saute" mode and cook the meal for 25 minutes.

**Nutrition value/serving:** calories 342, fat 14.2, fiber 1.1, carbs 6.6, protein 44.4

## Chicken Adobo

*Prep time: 10 minutes | Cooking time: 16 minutes | Servings: 2*

**Ingredients:**
- 4 chicken thighs
- 1 tablespoon apple cider vinegar
- ¼ teaspoon salt
- ½ teaspoon ground black pepper
- ½ cup water
- 1 teaspoon minced garlic

**Directions:**
Pour water in the instant pot bowl. Rub the chicken thighs with the salt, ground black pepper, and minced garlic. Let it marinade for 5 minutes. Then sprinkle the chicken with the apple cider vinegar. Place the chicken in the instant pot bowl and saute it for 2 minutes from each side. Then add water and close the instant pot bowl. Set the "Manual" mode (High pressure – natural release). Turn on the timer for 12 minutes. Serve the chicken with gravy!

**Nutrition value/serving:** calories 325, fat 20, fiber 0.2, carbs 0.9, protein 38.2

## Beef Bowl

*Prep time: 10 minutes | Cooking time: 30 minutes | Servings: 2*

**Ingredients:**
- 15 oz beef loin, chopped
- 1 tablespoon fresh cilantro, chopped
- 1 cup water
- ½ white onion
- ½ teaspoon ground coriander
- ½ teaspoon turmeric
- 1/3 teaspoon ground black pepper
- ½ teaspoon salt
- 1 teaspoon butter

**Directions:**
Pour water in the instant pot bowl. Add chopped beef loin, fresh cilantro, ground coriander, turmeric, ground black pepper, and butter. Cut the onion into halves and add in the beef mixture. Close the instant pot lid and set "Meat" mode. Cook the meat for 30 minutes – to get the soft taste (reduce the time if you prefer medium-rare meat)

**Nutrition value/serving:** calories 347, fat 17.2, fiber 0.8, carbs 5.7, protein 39.6

# Fragrant Taco Meat

*Prep time:* 5 *minutes* | *Cooking time:* 11 *minutes* | *Servings:* 2

**Ingredients:**

- 1 teaspoon Taco seasoning
- 9 oz ground beef
- 1 tomato, chopped
- ¼ cup water
- ½ teaspoon salt
- ½ teaspoon ground black pepper

**Directions:**

Place the ground beef and chopped tomato in the instant pot bowl. Start to saute the meat. Cook it for 5 minutes. After this, and Taco seasoning, salt, and ground black pepper. Stir it well. Add water and close the lid. Set the "Manual" mode (High pressure) and cook the meat for 6 minutes more. After this, use the quick pressure release method and transfer the meat in the serving bowls.

**Nutrition value/serving:** calories 249, fat 8, fiber 0.5, carbs 2.6, protein 39

# Shredded Pot Roast

*Prep time:* 15 *minutes* | *Cooking time:* 20 *minutes* | *Servings:* 2

**Ingredients:**

- 16 oz chuck roast
- 1 teaspoon rosemary
- ½ teaspoon coriander
- ½ teaspoon salt
- 1 carrot, chopped
- 1 cup water
- ½ teaspoon cayenne pepper

**Directions:**

Chop the chuck roast roughly and rub the meat with the rosemary, coriander, salt, and cayenne pepper. Preheat the instant pot on "Saute" mode, when the instant pot is hot – place the chuck roast inside. Cook it for 3 minutes. After this, add chopped carrot and water. Close the instant pot lid and seal it. Set the "Meat" mode and cook it for 20 minutes. Let the cooked meat rest for 5-10 minutes.

**Nutrition value/serving:** calories 506, fat 19, fiber 1.1, carbs 3.6, protein 75.2

# Beef Stew

*Prep time: 10 minutes | **Cooking time:** 39 minutes | **Servings:** 2*

## Ingredients:

- 9 oz beef sirloin, chopped
- 6 oz white mushrooms, sliced
- 1 tablespoon fresh cilantro, chopped
- 1 garlic clove, crushed
- ½ teaspoon salt
- 1 green pepper, chopped
- 1 cup water

## Directions:

Preheat the instant pot on "Saute" mode. When the title "Hot" is displayed – add chopped sirloin and cook it for 4 minutes (for 2 minutes from each side). Then add the crushed garlic clove, salt, chopped green pepper, cilantro, and mushrooms. Add water and close the instant pot lid. Saute the stew for 35 minutes – to get the tender taste.

**Nutrition value/serving:** calories 269, fat 8.3, fiber 1.9, carbs 6.1, protein 42

# Shrimp Soup

*Prep time: 5 minutes | **Cooking time:** 8 minutes | **Servings:** 2*

## Ingredients:

- 1 cup water
- ¼ cup coconut milk
- ½ green pepper, chopped
- ¼ white onion, diced
- 1 teaspoon turmeric
- ½ teaspoon ground red pepper
- ½ teaspoon salt
- 7 oz shrimps, peeled
- 1 teaspoon cilantro

## Directions:

Set "Saute" mode at instant pot. When the "Hot" is displayed – pour water and coconut milk inside instant pot bowl. Add turmeric, ground red pepper, salt, and cilantro. When the liquid start to boil – add diced onion, green pepper, and peeled shrimps. Close the lid and change the "Saute" mode into "Manual" (High pressure). Set the timer on 4 minutes. When the time is over – use the quick pressure release method. Ladle the soup into the bowls and serve it hot!

**Nutrition value/serving:** calories 489, fat 13.4, fiber 1, carbs 7, protein 79.4

## Stuffed Chicken Breast

*Prep time: 15 minutes | Cooking time: 15 minutes | Servings: 2*

**Ingredients:**

- 12 oz chicken breast, boneless, skinless
- 5 oz bacon, sliced
- 1 tablespoon cream cheese
- ½ teaspoon cayenne pepper
- ½ teaspoon ground white pepper
- ½ teaspoon minced garlic
- 1 teaspoon salt
- ¾ cup blackberries
- 1 tablespoon butter
- ¾ cup water

**Directions:**

Whisk together the cream cheese, cayenne pepper, ground white pepper, minced garlic, and salt. Then beat the chicken breast with the help of the kitchen hammer gently. It will make the final taste of meat tender and juicy. After this, spread the inside part of the chicken breast with the cream cheese mixture. Add blackberries and butter. Roll up the chicken breast to make the roll. Wrap the chicken breast into sliced bacon. Secure the chicken roll with the help of the kitchen twine. Wrap the roll into the foil. Pour 1 cup of water in the instant pot bowl and place the trivet. Place the chicken roll on the trivet and close the lid. Set the "Steam" mode and High pressure. Cook the chicken roll for 15 minutes. Then use the natural pressure release method. Slice the chicken roll.

**Nutrition value/serving:** calories 673, fat 41.7, fiber 3.1, carbs 7.2, protein 63.7

## Keto Chili

*Prep time: 5 minutes | Cooking time: 15 minutes | Servings: 2*

**Ingredients:**

- 13 oz ground beef
- 1 green chili pepper, chopped
- ½ white onion, diced
- ½ teaspoon ground black pepper
- ½ teaspoon ground cumin
- ½ teaspoon salt
- ¾ teaspoon chili powder
- 1 tomato, chopped
- ½ teaspoon minced garlic
- 1/3 cup water

**Directions:**

Preheat the instant pot bowl on "Saute" mode until it is displayed "Hot". Then place the ground beef there. Sprinkle it with the ground black pepper, cumin, chili powder, minced garlic, and salt. Stir gently and saute for 4 minutes. After this, add the chopped tomato and green chili pepper. Add water and close the lid. Saute the chili for 10 minutes. When the chili is cooked – transfer it directly into the serving bowls.

**Nutrition value/serving:** calories 367, fat 11.9, fiber 1.6, carbs 5.3, protein 56.8

## Buffalo Chicken

*Prep time: 7 minutes | **Cooking time:** 5 minutes | **Servings:** 2*

**Ingredients:**
- 10 oz chicken fillet
- ¾ cup almond flour
- 1 egg, whisked
- ½ teaspoon salt
- 1 tablespoon almond milk
- 1 tablespoon olive oil
- ¼ teaspoon ground black pepper
- Keto buffalo sauce (if desired)

**Directions:**

Cut the chicken fillet into the medium strips. Rub the chicken with the salt and ground black pepper. After this, dip the chicken strips into the almond flour. Stir together the almond milk and whisked the egg. Sip the chicken strips into the egg mixture. Pour olive oil in the instant pot bowl. Transfer the chicken strips into the instant pot, lock the lid and seal. Set the "Manual" mode and High pressure and cook the chicken for 5 minutes. Make a quick pressure release and serve the chicken hot!

**Nutrition value/serving:** calories 573, fat 36.6, fiber 4.7, carbs 9.8, protein 53

## Pork Carnitas

*Prep time: 8 minutes | **Cooking time:** 50 minutes | **Servings:** 2*

**Ingredients:**
- 11 oz pork shoulder, boneless
- ¼ teaspoon ground cumin
- ½ teaspoon salt
- 1 teaspoon dried oregano
- 2 tablespoons butter
- ¼ teaspoon white pepper
- ½ cup water

**Directions:**

Rub the pork shoulder with the ground cumin, salt, dried oregano, and white pepper carefully. Place the pork shoulder in the instant pot and add water. Seal the instant pot lid and set the "Manual" mode (High pressure). Set timer for 40 minutes. When the time is running out – make the natural pressure release for 10 minutes. Then chop the meat and sprinkle with the remaining gravy.

**Nutrition value/serving:** calories 561, fat 45, fiber 0.4, carbs 0.8, protein 36.6

# Spicy Chicken Drumsticks
*Prep time: 10 minutes | Cooking time: 15 minutes | Servings: 2*

## Ingredients:
- ½ teaspoon cayenne pepper
- ½ teaspoon chili flakes
- ¼ teaspoon ground black pepper
- ½ teaspoon dried basil
- 4 drumstick
- ¼ cup full-fat cream
- 1 teaspoon butter

## Directions:
Mix up together the cayenne pepper, chili flakes, ground black pepper, and dried basil. Rub the chicken drumstick with the spice mixture evenly. Melt the butter and mix it up with the full-fat cream. Place the chicken drumstick on the foil and sprinkle with the creamy liquid. Pour 1 cup of water in the instant pot and place the trivet there. Wrap the chicken drumsticks in the foil carefully and transfer on the instant pot trivet. Lock the instant pot lid and seal it. Set the "Poultry" mode and timer for 15 minutes (High pressure). When the poultry is cooked – use the quick pressure release method. Discard the foil from the drumstick.

**Nutrition value/serving:** calories 210, fat 10.5, fiber 0.2, carbs 1.8, protein 25.9

# Beef Stroganoff
*Prep time: 6 minutes | Cooking time: 20 minutes | Servings: 2*

## Ingredients:
- 1 teaspoon dried basil
- ½ teaspoon salt
- 14 oz beef brisket
- 4 oz white mushrooms, chopped
- ½ cup water
- ½ teaspoon ground black pepper
- 1 teaspoon butter
- 1 tablespoon cream cheese

## Directions:
Preheat the instant pot on "Saute" mode. When it is displayed "hot" – toss the butter inside and melt it. Chop the beef brisket and add in the melted butter. Sprinkle the meat with the ground black pepper and dried basil. Saute it for 5 minutes. Stir it once per cooking time. Then add chopped mushrooms, cream cheese, and water. Stir gently and close the lid. Seal the lid and set the "manual" mode. Put the timer on 15 minutes (High Pressure). When the time is over – make the quick pressure release according to the directions of your instant pot. Place the cooked beef stroganoff on the plates.

**Nutrition value/serving:** calories 417, fat 16.2, fiber 0.7, carbs 2.3, protein 62.5

# Pork Chops

*Prep time: 5 minutes | Cooking time: 12 minutes | Servings: 2*

## Ingredients:

- 13 oz pork chops
- 1 teaspoon ground black pepper
- 1 teaspoon salt
- 1 cup water
- ½ onion

## Directions:

Rub the pork chops with the ground black pepper and salt. Place the pork chops in the instant pot. Add water and onion. Lock the instant pot lid and set "meat" mode (High Pressure). Cook pork chops for 12 minutes + quick pressure release.

**Nutrition value/serving:** calories 603, fat 45.9, fiber 0.9, carbs 3.3, protein 41.8

# Salmon Cutlets

*Prep time: 10 minutes | Cooking time: 4 minutes | Servings: 2*

## Ingredients:

- 1 tablespoon dried dill
- 10 oz salmon fillet
- ½ teaspoon minced garlic
- ¼ teaspoon minced ginger
- ½ teaspoon salt
- 1 tablespoon butter
- 1 tablespoon almond flour
- 1 small egg, whisked

## Directions:

Rind the salmon fillet and combine it together with the minced garlic, minced ginger, dried dill, salt, and whisked the egg. Stir until homogenous. Then make the small cutlets from the fish mixture and sprinkle them with the almond flour. Preheat the instant pot on the "Saute" mode until it is displayed "Hot". Toss the butter inside and melt it. Transfer the salmon cutlets in the instant pot and cook them for 2 minutes from each side.

**Nutrition value/serving:** calories 351, fat 23.4, fiber 1.8, carbs 4.4, protein 33.3

# Chicken Kebab with Green Pepper
*Prep time: 10 minutes | Cooking time: 5 minutes | Servings: 2*

**Ingredients:**
- 1 green pepper
- 1 tablespoon lemon juice
- ½ teaspoon cayenne pepper
- ½ teaspoon salt
- 10 oz chicken fillet
- 1 tablespoon olive oil

**Directions:**
Cut the green pepper into the medium squares. Chop the fillet into the medium cubes. Place together the green pepper squares and chicken cubes. Sprinkle the ingredients with the lemon juice, cayenne pepper, salt, and olive oil. Let it marinate for 10 minutes. After this, string the ingredients on the skewers. Place them in the cake mold. Pour 1 cup of water in the instant pot and place trivet. Transfer the cake mold in the instant pot, on the trivet. Sprinkle the kebabs with the remaining oil mixture. Lock the instant pot lid and set "Manual" mode (High Pressure). Set timer for 5 minutes. After this, make a quick pressure release.

**Nutrition value/serving:** calories 344, fat 17.7, fiber 1.2, carbs 3.2, protein 41.6

# Parmesan Chicken Cubes
*Prep time: 10 minutes | Cooking time: 15 minutes | Servings: 2*

**Ingredients:**
- 2 oz Parmesan, grated
- 10 oz chicken breast, skinless, boneless
- 1 teaspoon dried rosemary
- 1 tablespoon butter
- ¾ cup heavy cream
- ½ teaspoon salt
- ½ teaspoon red hot pepper

**Directions:**
Chop the chicken breast into the cubes. Toss butter in the instant pot and preheat it on "Saute" mode. Add the chicken cubes. Sprinkle the poultry with the dried rosemary, salt, and red hot pepper. Add cream and mix up together all the ingredients. Close the lid of the instant pot and seal it. Set "Poultry" mode and put a timer on 15 minutes. When the time is over – let the chicken rest for 5 minutes more. Transfer the meal on the plates and sprinkle with the grated cheese. The cheese shouldn't melt immediately.

**Nutrition value/serving:** calories 461, fat 32.1, fiber 0.3, carbs 2.7, protein 40.2

## Juicy Chopped Pork

*Prep time: 8 minutes | **Cooking time:** 30 minutes | **Servings:** 2*

**Ingredients:**

- 1 teaspoon apple cider vinegar
- 10 oz pork loin, chopped
- ½ cup water
- 1 oz carrot, chopped
- 1 teaspoon salt
- ½ teaspoon peppercorns

**Directions:**

Sprinkle the chopped pork loin with the apple cider vinegar. Then strew the meat with the salt. Place the meat in the mat mold. Insert the meat mold in the instant pot. Add water, carrot, and peppercorns. Close the lid and lock it. Set the "Meat" mode and put a timer on 30 minutes. When the meat is cooked – chill it till the room temperature.

**Nutrition value/serving:** calories 351, fat 19.8, fiber 0.5, carbs 1.8, protein 38.9

## Butter Beef

*Prep time: 10 minutes | **Cooking time:** 60 minutes | **Servings:** 2*

**Ingredients:**

- 10 oz beef arm roast
- 4 tablespoons butter
- 1 white onion, diced
- ½ teaspoon cayenne pepper
- ½ teaspoon salt
- 1 teaspoon dried basil
- ½ cup water

**Directions:**

Place the butter in the instant pot and start to preheat it on "Saute" mode. Meanwhile, mix up together the cayenne pepper, salt, and dried basil. Rub the beef arm with the spices and transfer the meat in the melted butter. Add diced onion and water. Close the instant pot lid and lock it. Set the "Manual" mode and put a timer on 60 minutes (Low Pressure). When the meat is cooked – serve it immediately and store in the fridge up to 3 days.

**Nutrition value/serving:** calories 533, fat 3, fiber 1.3, carbs 5.4, protein 47.7

# Spicy Meatloaf

*Prep time: 10 minutes | Cooking time: 10 minutes | Servings: 2*

## Ingredients:

- 10 oz ground beef
- 1 egg
- 1 tablespoon almond meal
- ½ teaspoon salt
- 1 teaspoon smoked paprika
- 1 tablespoon cream cheese
- 3 tablespoons water
- 1 teaspoon ground black pepper
- ¾ teaspoon cayenne pepper
- 1 teaspoon dried basil
- 1 teaspoon dried oregano
- 1 teaspoon dried parsley

## Directions:

Beat the egg in the bowl and whisk it. Add ground beef, almond meal, salt, smoked paprika, cream cheese, water, ground black pepper, cayenne pepper, dried basil, dried oregano, and dried parsley. Mix up together the mixture until homogenous. Take the loaf pan and place the meat mixture there. Flatten it well to make the shape of the meatloaf. Pour 1 cup of water in the instant pot. Insert the trivet in the instant pot and place the meatloaf pan on it. Cook the meal on High pressure for 10 minutes. Then make a quick pressure release. Chill the meatloaf little, slice it.

**Nutrition value/serving:** calories 340, fat 14.6, fiber 1.6, carbs 3.1, protein 47.2


# Seabass with Parmesan

*Prep time: 8 minutes | Cooking time: 4 minutes | Servings: 2*

## Ingredients:

- 10 oz seabass steak
- ¾ teaspoon dried thyme
- 1 tablespoon apple cider vinegar
- 1 oz Parmesan, grated
- ½ oz walnuts, crushed
- 1 tablespoon butter
- ½ teaspoon salt
- ¼ teaspoon cayenne pepper

## Directions:

Cut the seabass steak into halves. Sprinkle every seabass part with the dried thyme, apple cider vinegar, butter, salt, and cayenne pepper. Pour 1/2cup of water in the instant pot. Add butter and walnuts. Place the fish in the instant pot and close the lid. Cook the fish on High pressure for 4 minutes (Quick pressure release). Then sprinkle the cooked seabass with the grated cheese.

**Nutrition value/serving:** calories 244, fat 14.1, fiber 0.7, carbs 1.7, protein 29.4

## Cream Pork Liver

*Prep time: 5 minutes | Cooking time: 7 minutes | Servings: 2*

**Ingredients:**

- 14 oz pork liver, chopped
- ½ cup heavy cream
- ½ teaspoon salt
- ½ teaspoon ground black pepper
- ¾ teaspoon ground nutmeg
- 1 teaspoon butter

**Directions:**

Sprinkle the liver with the salt, ground black pepper, and nutmeg. Toss the butter in the instant pot and melt it on "Saute" mode. Add heavy cream and liver. Stir gently and close the lid. Cook the meal on "Saute" mode for 6 minutes.

**Nutrition value/serving:** calories 631, fat 48.6, fiber 0.3, carbs 1.6, protein 44.4

## Stuffed Eggplants

*Prep time: 15 minutes | Cooking time: 5 minutes | Servings: 2*

**Ingredients:**

- 1 eggplant
- 10 oz ground pork
- ½ teaspoon minced garlic
- 1 teaspoon ground black pepper
- ½ teaspoon salt
- 1 tablespoon butter
- 2 bacon slices

**Directions:**

Cut the eggplant into halves. Then remove ½ of pulp from the eggplants. Mix up together the minced garlic, ground black pepper. Salt, and ground pork. Fill the eggplants with the pork mixture. Cover the eggplant halves with the butter and bacon slices. Wrap the eggplants into the foil and transfer them on the steamer rack in the instant pot. Pour 1 cup of water in the instant pot and close the lid. Cook the eggplants on High Pressure (Steam mode) for 7 minutes. Then make the natural pressure release for 5 minutes. Discard the foil from the vegetables or serve it in the foil (make the shape of boats).

**Nutrition value/serving:** calories 417, fat 19.1, fiber 8.4, carbs 14.7, protein 46.6

# Garlic Beef Stew

*Prep time:* 10 minutes | *Cooking time:* 15 minutes | *Servings:* 2

## Ingredients:

- 3 garlic cloves
- ½ cup water
- ¼ cup heavy cream
- 14 oz beef sirloin, chopped
- 1 teaspoon salt
- 1 tablespoon fresh cilantro, chopped
- ½ teaspoon cayenne pepper
- ½ cup broccoli, chopped

## Directions:

Peel the garlic cloves and cut them into 3 parts. Pour water and heavy cream in the instant pot. Add garlic, salt, fresh cilantro, cayenne pepper, and chopped broccoli. Add beef sirloin and close the lid. Cook the meal on "Manual' mode (High pressure) for 15 minutes. Use the quick pressure release. Serve the stew when it reaches room temperature.

**Nutrition value/serving:** calories 363, fat 19.9, fiber 0.8, carbs 6.1, protein 37.9

# Desserts Recipes

## Pumpkin Pie Pudding
*Prep time: 10 minutes | Cooking time: 30 minutes | Servings: 2*

**Ingredients:**
- 1 egg, beaten
- ¼ cup heavy cream
- 1 tablespoon Splenda
- 3 tablespoons pumpkin puree
- ¼ teaspoon pumpkin pie spices
- 1 teaspoon butter
- 1 cup of water (for instant pot)

**Directions:**
Whisk the egg and mix it up with the heavy cream. Add Splenda, pumpkin puree, and pumpkin pie spices. Stir the mixture. Grease the cake pan with the butter and transfer the pumpkin mixture inside. Pour 1 cup of water in the instant pot. Insert the steam rack in the instant pot. Cover the pudding with the foil and secure edges. Insert the cake pan on the steam rack. Put the "Manual" mode (High pressure) for 20 minutes. When the time is over – make the natural pressure release for 10 minutes. Chill the pudding for 8 hours.

**Nutrition value/serving:** calories 116, fat 9.7, fiber 0.5, carbs 4, protein 3.3

## Brownie in Cup
*Prep time: 8 minutes | Cooking time: 10 minutes | Servings: 2*

**Ingredients:**
- ¼ cup sugar-free chocolate chips
- 1 egg, whisked
- 2 tablespoons butter
- 1 teaspoon Splenda
- 1 tablespoon almond flour
- ¼ teaspoon vanilla extract
- 1 cup of water (for instant pot)

**Directions:**
Mix up together the chocolate chips. Whisked egg, Splenda, almond flour, and vanilla extract. Melt the butter and add it in the mixture. Stir the mass until homogenous. Then transfer the liquid into the medium cups (ramekins). Pour 1 cup of water in the instant pot. Place the steamer rack. Transfer the cups on the steamer rack and close the lid. Seal the instant pot lid and set the "Manual" mode. Put the timer for 9 minutes (Quick pressure release). When the dessert is cooked – let it chill for 1 hour.

**Nutrition value/serving:** calories 186, fat 16.5, fiber 0.4, carbs 6.3, protein 3.8

# Coconut Bites

*Prep time: 5 minutes | Cooking time: 8 minutes | Servings: 2*

**Ingredients:**

- 2 tablespoon coconut flakes
- 1 egg, whisked
- 2 tablespoons almond flour
- ¾ teaspoon vanilla extract
- 1 teaspoon swerve
- 1 tablespoon butter
- ¾ teaspoon baking powder
- 1 cup of water (for instant pot)

**Directions:**

Grease the ramekins with the butter generously. After this, combine together the whisked egg, almond flour, coconut flakes, and vanilla extract in the separated bowl. Add baking powder and swerve. Stir the mixture well. Place the mixture into the prepared ramekins. Fill ¼ part of every ramekin. Pour 1 cup of water in the instant pot. Insert the steamer rack inside and place the ramekins on it. Close and lock the instant pot lid. Set the "Manual" mode for 8 minutes – high Pressure. When the time is over – make the quick pressure release for 5 minutes. Chill the dessert for 5-10 minutes or until they are warm. Remove the coconut bites from the ramekins.

**Nutrition value/serving:** calories 148, fat 13, fiber 1.2, carbs 7, protein 4.5

# Keto Mousse

*Prep time: 6 minutes | Cooking time: 8 minutes | Servings: 2*

**Ingredients:**

- 2 egg yolks, whisked
- 2 tablespoons Erythritol
- 1 teaspoon vanilla extract
- 1 tablespoon coconut flour
- 4 tablespoon heavy cream
- 2 tablespoon almond milk
- 1 cup of water (for instant pot)

**Directions:**

Place the whisked egg yolks in the instant pot bowl and start to saute them for 3 minutes. Stir them all the time. Then start to add heavy cream gradually. When the mixture is homogenous – add vanilla extract, coconut flour, and almond milk. Stir it until smooth. Add Erythritol ad stir well. After this, pour the mixture into the medium jars. Pour 1 cup of water in the instant pot and insert the steamer rack. Place the jars with mousse on the rack and close the lid. Seal the instant pot lid and set the "Manual" mode for 5 minutes (High Pressure). When the time is over – make a quick pressure release. Remove the jars with mousse from the instant pot and let them chill for 5 hours in the fridge.

**Nutrition value/serving:** calories 228, fat 19.9, fiber 3.3, carbs 7.6, protein 4.7

## Soft Keto Cheesecake

*Prep time: 10 minutes | **Cooking time:** 30 minutes | **Servings:** 2*

**Ingredients:**
- 4 tablespoon cream cheese
- 1 tablespoon swerve
- ¾ teaspoon vanilla extract
- 1 egg, whisked
- 2 tablespoon heavy cream
- 1 teaspoon coconut flakes
- 1 cup of water (for instant pot)

**Directions:**

Mix up together the whisked egg and cream cheese. Add vanilla extract, heavy cream, and swerve. Use the hand mixer to make the smooth and fluffy mass. When the mass is soft and fluffy – pour it into the cake mold. Pour 1 cup of water in the instant pot. Insert the trivet. Place the cheesecake on the trivet. Close and seal the instant pot lid. Cook the cheesecake on "manual" mode for 30 minutes (High pressure). Then make the natural pressure release for 10 minutes. Let the cooked dessert chill well. Cut it into the servings.

**Nutrition value/serving:** calories 195, fat 18, fiber 0.2, carbs 4.4, protein 5

## Carrot Cake Cups

*Prep time: 15 minutes | **Cooking time:** 10 minutes | **Servings:** 2*

**Ingredients:**
- 1 egg
- 1 tablespoon butter
- 1 teaspoon liquid stevia
- ¾ teaspoon vanilla extract
- 2 tablespoon carrot, grated
- 1 tablespoon walnuts, crushed
- ¾ cup almond flour
- ¾ teaspoon ground ginger
- ¾ teaspoon baking powder
- 1 cup of water (for instant pot)

**Directions:**

Beat the egg in the mixing bowl and whisk it well with the help of the hand whisker. Add liquid stevia, vanilla extract, almond flour. Ground ginger, and baking powder. Stir well until smooth. Then add walnuts and grated carrot. Mix up the batter with the help of the spoon until homogenous. Pour the batter into the non-sticky cake mold. Then pour 1 cup of water in the instant pot. Insert the steamer rack. Transfer the cake on the rack and close the instant pot lid. Seal the lid and set the "Manual" mode (High pressure) for 10 minutes. Use the quick pressure release method when the cake is cooked. Chill the cake for 10-15 minutes. Cut it into servings.

**Nutrition value/serving:** calories 128, fat 11.1, fiber 0.8 carbs 3.2, protein 4.3

## Creme Brulee

*Prep time:* 10 minutes | *Cooking time:* 9 minutes | *Servings:* 2

### Ingredients:

- 1 cup heavy cream
- 3 egg yolks
- 2 teaspoons Erythritol
- ½ teaspoon vanilla extract
- 1 cup of water (for instant pot)

### Directions:

Whisk the egg yolk until you get the yellow color. Then add heavy cream and keep whisking the egg yolk mixture until smooth. Add 1 teaspoon of Erythritol and vanilla extract. Stir it well and transfer into the ramekins. Pour 1 cup of water in the instant pot bowl. Place the steamer rack inside the instant pot. Transfer the ramekins on the rack and wrap the top of ramekins with the foil. Close the lid and seal it. Set the "Manual" mode (High pressure) and cook the dessert for 9 minutes. After this, make the natural pressure release for 15 minutes. Chill the dessert for 2 hours. After this, sprinkle the top of the ramekins with the remaining Erythritol and burn the sweetener with the help of the hand torch.

**Nutrition value/serving:** calories 291, fat 29, fiber 0, carbs 2.7, protein 5.3

## Blackberry Muffins

*Prep time:* 15 minutes | *Cooking time:* 14 minutes | *Servings:* 2

### Ingredients:

- 2 tablespoons almond flour
- 1 teaspoon flax meal
- 2 teaspoon swerve
- ¼ teaspoon baking powder
- 3 tablespoons almond milk
- 1 egg, beaten
- 1 teaspoon butter
- 1 oz blackberries
- 1 cup of water (for instant pot)

### Directions:

Whisk together the beaten egg, butter, almond milk, and baking powder. Add swerve and flax meal. After this, add almond flour and stir until homogenous. Add the blackberries and stir the batter with the help of a spoon. Pour the butter into the muffin molds. Pour 1 cup of water in the instant pot and insert the steamer ramekin. Transfer the muffins on the rack and wrap them in foil. Set the "Manual" mode and put the timer on 14 minutes (High Pressure – QR for 10 minutes). Chill the muffins until warm.

**Nutrition value/serving:** calories 120, fat 10.7, fiber 1.8, carbs 8.7, protein 4.1

## Keto Brownies

*Prep time: 20 minutes | Cooking time: 10 minutes | Servings: 2*

- 2 tablespoons almond milk
- 2 oz dark chocolate, chopped
- 1 tablespoon Erythritol
- ¼ teaspoon vanilla extract
- 2 egg yolks, whisked
- ¼ cup heavy cream
- 1 teaspoon butter
- 3 tablespoon almond flour, gluten-free
- 1 cup of water (for instant pot)

**Directions:**

Pour almond milk in the instant pot bowl and start to cook it on "saute" mode. Add chopped dark chocolate and vanilla extract. Add heavy cream and butter. When the mixture is smooth – start to add whisked egg yolks gradually. Add almond meal. Whisk the mixture without stopping. Add Erythritol and cook the meal for 3 minutes. Whisk it all the time. Then pour the chocolate mixture into the jars. Pour 1 cup of water in the instant pot. Place the trivet and put the jars on the trivet. Cook the dessert on "manual" mode for 10 minutes (QR for 5 minutes). Chill the brownies for 10 minutes and eat with the help of the teaspoon.

**Nutrition value/serving:** calories 334, fat 29, fiber 3.3, carbs 9.3, protein 4.6

## Lemon Curd

*Prep time: 5 minutes | Cooking time: 5 minutes | Servings: 2*

**Ingredients:**

- 3 egg yolks, whisked
- 2 tablespoon butter
- 6 drops liquid stevia
- ¼ cup lemon juice
- ¾ teaspoon lemon zest, grated

**Directions:**

Set the instant pot in "Saute" mode and when the "Hot" is displayed – add butter. Melt the butter but not boil it and add whisked egg yolks and lemon juice. Add stevia and lemon zest. Whisk the mixture. Saute the curd for 3 minutes on "Saute" mode. Then whisk the lemon curd until smooth and transfer in the serving ramekins. Chill it well.

**Nutrition value/serving:** calories 190, fat 18.5, fiber 0.2, carbs 1.7, protein 4.4

# Pudding Cake

*Prep time: 15 minutes | Cooking time: 10 minutes | Servings: 2*

## Ingredients:

- ¼ teaspoon baking powder
- 4 tablespoon almond flour
- 1 teaspoon coconut flour
- 1 tablespoon cocoa powder
- 1 tablespoon Erythritol
- 1 egg, whisked
- ½ cup coconut milk
- 1/3 teaspoon ground cinnamon
- 1 cup of water (for instant pot)

## Directions:

Mix up together all the dry ingredients. Then add all the liquid ingredients and stir carefully until homogenous. Pour 1 cup of water in the instant pot and insert trivet. Place the chocolate batter in the springform pan or cake pan (non-sticky) and transfer on the trivet. Cover the top of the pan with the foil and close the instant pot lid. Cook the meal on "Manual" mode for 10 minutes (High pressure). Then use the quick pressure release for 5 minutes. Let the cooked pudding chill till the room temperature.

**Nutrition value/serving:** calories 268, fat 24, fiber 5.2, carbs 10.4, protein 7.9

# Mug Cake

*Prep time: 10 minutes | Cooking time: 8 minutes | Servings: 2*

## Ingredients:

- 1 teaspoon olive oil
- 2 tablespoon almond flour
- 2 eggs, beaten
- 1 tablespoon Erythritol
- ½ teaspoon vanilla extract
- ¼ teaspoon baking powder
- 1 tablespoon butter
- 1 cup of water (for instant pot)

## Directions:

Spread the mugs with the olive oil. Mix up together all remaining the liquid ingredients and butter. Add all the dry ingredients and stir the mixture with the help of the spoon. When you get smooth batter – transfer it into the prepared mugs. Pour 1 cup of water in the instant pot and insert the steamer rack. Put the nugs on the rack and close the lid. Cook the meal on "Manual" (High pressure) for 8 minutes. Then make the quick pressure release for 5 minutes. Let the cooked mug cakes chill for 3-5 minutes.

**Nutrition value/serving:** calories 174, fat 15.7, fiber 0.7, carbs 2.1, protein 6.8

# Almond Slices

*Prep time:* 20 minutes | *Cooking time:* 8 minutes | *Servings:* 2

## Ingredients:
- 1 oz almonds, crushed
- 1 tablespoon butter, softened
- 1 egg, whisked
- ½ cup almond flour
- 1 tablespoon Erythritol
- ½ teaspoon vanilla extract
- ¼ cup almond milk
- ¾ teaspoon ground cinnamon
- ½ teaspoon olive oil

## Directions:
Spread the non-sticky springform mold with the olive oil. Then combine together the softened butter, whisked egg, almond flour, vanilla extract, almond milk, Erythritol, and ground cinnamon. Check if all the ingredients are added and mix up the mixture until smooth. Transfer the mixture in the prepared springform pan and flatten it well. Place the pan in the instant pot and cover with the foil. Close the lid and cook the dessert on "Manual" mode for 8 minutes (follow the directions of your instant pot). Then make the natural pressure release for 15 minutes. Chill the cooked dessert well and cut it into the slices.

**Nutrition value/serving:** calories 283, fat 26.4, fiber 3.6, carbs 6.7, protein 7.8

# Cardamom Tender Cake

*Prep time:* 15 minutes | *Cooking time:* 10 minutes | *Servings:* 2

## Ingredients:
- 1 teaspoon ground cardamom
- ½ teaspoon ground cinnamon
- 1 egg, whisked
- 1/3 teaspoon baking powder
- ¼ teaspoon vanilla extract
- ½ cup almond flour
- 1 tablespoon butter
- ¼ cup water
- ½ cup water (for instant pot)

## Directions:
Stir together the whisked egg and water. Add butter, almond flour, vanilla extract, baking powder, ground cinnamon, and ground cardamom. Stir the mixture together until smooth and homogenous. Transfer the dough into the non-sticky cake pan and flatten it well with the help of the fingertips. Pour ½ cup of water in the instant pot bowl and insert the trivet. Put the cake pan on the trivet and cover it with the foil. Close and seal the lid. Set the "Manual" mode (High pressure) for 10 minutes. Then make natural pressure release according to the directions of your instant pot. Cut the cake into the servings. Serve with the whipped cream, if desired.

**Nutrition value/serving:** calories 237, fat 21.1, fiber 3.3, carbs 6.9, protein 7.9

## Chocolate Cake

*Prep time: 12 minutes | Cooking time: 13 minutes | Servings: 2*

**Ingredients:**

- 1 teaspoon ground ginger
- ¼ teaspoon vanilla extract
- 1 tablespoon butter
- ½ cup almond milk
- 4 tablespoon almond flour
- 1 tablespoon cocoa powder
- 1 tablespoon Erythritol
- ¼ teaspoon olive oil
- 1 cup of water (for instant pot)

**Directions:**

Spread the springform pan with the olive oil. Mix up together all the dry ingredients. Then mix up together all the liquid ingredients. Combine together dry and liquid ingredients and stir carefully with the help of the spoon. When you get smooth mixture – place it in the springform pan and flatten the surface with the help of a spatula. Pour 1 cup of water in the instant pot bowl and insert the trivet. Transfer the springform pan on the trivet and cover the top with the foil. Secure the edges of the springform pan with the foil. Close and seal the instant pot lid. Set the "Manual" mode and put the timer on 13 minutes. When the time is over – use the quick pressure release method (5 minutes). Chill the cake till the room temperature and slice it.

**Nutrition value/serving:** calories 303, fat 29.8, fiber 4.1, carbs 8.9, protein 5.3

## Cinnamon Roll

*Prep time: 20 minutes | Cooking time: 18 minutes | Servings: 2*

**Ingredients:**

- ½ cup almond flour
- 1 tablespoon ground cinnamon
- 2 tablespoon Erythritol
- 1 egg, whisked
- ¼ cup almond milk
- 1 tablespoon butter, softened
- 1/3 cup of water (for instant pot)

**Directions:**

Combine together almond flour, almond milk, and softened butter. Knead the smooth dough. Roll up the dough with the help of the rolling pin. Then combine together Erythritol and ground cinnamon. Sprinkle the surface of the dough with the ground cinnamon mixture generously. Roll the dough into one big roll. Place the roll into the instant pot round mold. Pour water in the instant pot (1/3 cup) and insert the mold inside. Set "Manual" mode (High pressure) for 18 minutes. Then use the natural pressure release method for 15 minutes. Chill the roll till the room temperature and cut into the halves.

**Nutrition value/serving:** calories 455, fat 41.2, fiber 7.9, carbs 14.8, protein 13.6

# Lava Cake

*Prep time: 15 minutes | **Cooking time:** 4 minutes | **Servings:** 2*

**Ingredients:**

- 1 oz dark chocolate, sugar-free
- ¼ teaspoon vanilla extract
- 3 eggs, whisked
- 3 tablespoon butter
- ½ teaspoon baking powder
- ½ teaspoon lemon juice
- 4 tablespoons almond flour

**Directions:**

Melt the dark chocolate until liquid. Add vanilla extract and butter. Whisk it well. After this, add whisked eggs, lemon juice, baking powder, and almond flour. Stir the mixture with the help of the fork until smooth texture. Pour the chocolate batter into 2 small cake molds. Place the trivet in the instant pot and add water in the bottom. Add the cake molds and close the lid. Set "Manual" mode for 4 minutes (High pressure). When the time is over – use the natural pressure release method for 10 minutes.

**Nutrition value/serving:** calories 437, fat 40.4, fiber 3.6, carbs 8.2, protein 14.5

# Pumpkin Cheesecake

*Prep time: 6 minutes | **Cooking time:** 15 minutes | **Servings:** 2*

**Ingredients:**

- 1 tablespoon pumpkin puree
- 2 tablespoon cream cheese
- 1 tablespoon Erythritol
- 1 teaspoon pumpkin pie spices
- 2 eggs, whisked
- 1 tablespoon coconut flour
- 1 cup water (for instant pot)

**Directions:**

Whisk the cream cheese with the help of the hand mixer until it is fluffy. After this, add Erythritol and pumpkin pie spices. Add pumpkin puree and whisked eggs. Add the coconut flour and whisk the mixture with the hand blender until smooth. Pour the mixture into the cheesecake mold and flatten gently. Pour 1 cup of water in the instant pot bowl and insert the trivet. Transfer the cheesecake mold on the trivet and close the lid. Set the "Steam" mode and cook the cheesecake for 15 minutes. Chill the dessert till the room temperature and cut into the servings.

**Nutrition value/serving:** calories 138, fat 9.7, fiber 2.9, carbs 6.3, protein 7.9

# Custard Cups

*Prep time: 10 minutes | Cooking time: 8 minutes | Servings: 2*

**Ingredients:**

- 1 cup almond milk
- 1 tablespoon almond flour
- 3 egg yolks
- 1 tablespoon Erythritol
- ½ teaspoon vanilla extract
- 1 tablespoon butter

**Directions:**

Whisk the egg yolks carefully. Add the almond milk into the egg yolks. After this, add Erythritol and vanilla extract. Stir the mixture and transfer it into the instant pot bowl. Start to saute the mixture on "Saute" mode. Cook the custard for 4 minutes. Stir it time to time. Then add almond flour. Stir it until homogenous. Cook it for 4 minutes more and stir constantly. Then add butter and mix up the mixture until smooth. Pour the cooked dessert into the serving glass cups and chill till the room temperature. Place the teaspoons inside the cups.

**Nutrition value/serving:** calories 434, fat 43.2, fiber 3.1, carbs 8.5, protein 7.7

# Lemon Cakes in Mug

*Prep time: 15 minutes | Cooking time: 15 minutes | Servings: 2*

**Ingredients:**

- ½ cup heavy cream
- ½ teaspoon lemon zest, grated
- 1/3 teaspoon baking powder
- 4 tablespoons coconut flour
- 1 egg yolk
- 1 tablespoon liquid stevia
- 1 cup water (for instant pot)

**Directions:**

Whisk the heavy cream gently and add lemon zest. Add baking powder and coconut flour. After this, whisk the egg and add it into the cream mixture. Add liquid stevia. Whisk the mixture until smooth and pour into the mugs or jars. Cover the top of the mugs with the foil and make the small holes with the help of the toothpick. Pour water into the instant pot and insert the steamer rack. Place the mugs on the steamer rack and close the lid. Seal the lid and set the "steam" mode. Cook the cakes for 13 minutes. After this, use the quick pressure release for 4 minutes. Chill the cakes for 5 minutes and discard the foil.

**Nutrition value/serving:** calories 191, fat 11.5, fiber 10.1, carbs 17.7, protein 7.4

# Sweet Blueberry Bread

*Prep time: 5 minutes | Cooking time: 3 minutes | Servings: 2*

**Ingredients:**
- ¼ cup fresh blueberries
- ½ teaspoon baking powder
- ¼ teaspoon lemon juice
- 1 teaspoon vanilla extract
- 1 tablespoon Erythritol
- 1 egg, whisked
- ¼ cup full-fat cream
- ½ cup almond flour
- 1 cup water (for instant pot)

**Directions:**

Mash the blueberries gently. Combine together the baking powder, lemon juice, vanilla extract, Erythritol, and whisked egg. Add full-fat cream and almond flour. Add blueberries. Mix up the mixture until you get the homogenous texture. Transfer the dough into the non-sticky cake mold and flatten gently with the help of the spatula. Wrap the mold in the aluminum foil. Pour water in the instant pot and insert the steamer rack. Place the mold on the rack and close the lid. Seal the instant pot lid and set "Steam" mode. Cook the sweet bread for 20 minutes. Then use the quick pressure release according to the directions of your instant pot). Chill the bread and remove it from the cake mold. Cut into servings.

**Nutrition value/serving:** calories 238, fat 18.9, fiber 3.1, carbs 10.8, protein 8.8

# Keto Apple-Free Crisps

*Prep time: 6 minutes | Cooking time: 8 minutes | Servings: 2*

**Ingredients:**
- 1 tablespoon almond flour
- 1 tablespoon Erythritol
- ½ teaspoon ground cinnamon
- ¼ teaspoon vanilla extract
- 1 zucchini
- 1 tablespoon butter

**Directions:**

Peel the zucchini and cut it into the cubes. Sprinkle the zucchini cubes with Erythritol and shake well to get the homogenous texture. Add ground cinnamon and sprinkle with the vanilla extract. Stir with the help of the big spoon. Toss the butter in the instant pot and melt it on "Saute" mode. Transfer the zucchini into the instant pot and stir well. Then sprinkle them with the almond flour and stir gently. Close the lid and saute the meal for 6 minutes. When the time is over – don't stir the dessert anymore and transfer directly into serving bowls.

**Nutrition value/serving:** calories 93, fat 8, fiber 1.8, carbs 4.6, protein 2.1

# Coconut Bars

*Prep time: 5 minutes | Cooking time: 5 minutes | Servings: 2*

### Ingredients:
- 2 tablespoons coconut flakes
- 5 tablespoon almond flour
- 5 drops liquid stevia
- ½ teaspoon vanilla extract
- 1 egg white, whisked
- 1 cup of water (for instant pot)

### Directions:
Combine together all the dry ingredients. Then add vanilla extract, liquid stevia, and whisked the egg. Stir the mixture until it is smooth. The dough shouldn't be liquid. Then place the dough into the springform pan and flatten it well with the help of the spoon. Pour 1 cup of water in the instant pot and place the trivet. Put the springform pan on the trivet and cover the top of it with the foil (it will prevent the crunchy surface). Then set "Manual" mode (High Pressure) for 5 minutes. When the time is over – make a quick pressure release. Chill the dessert till the warm temperature and cut it into the bars.

**Nutrition value/serving:** calories 209, fat 16.7, fiber 3.5, carbs 6, protein 9

# Keto Hot Chocolate

*Prep time: 2 minutes | Cooking time: 7 minutes | Servings: 2*

### Ingredients:
- 1 cup almond milk
- 3 tablespoon full-fat cream
- 1 teaspoon butter
- ½ teaspoon ground cinnamon
- 1 teaspoon erythritol
- 1 oz dark chocolate

### Directions:
Transfer all the ingredients into the instant pot bowl. Set the "Saute" and start to cook the hot chocolate. Stir well. Saute the hot chocolate until it starts to boil. (around 5-7 minutes). Pour the dessert into the cups.

**Nutrition value/serving:** calories 381, fat 35.9, fiber 3.9, carbs 8.7, protein 3.6

# Keto Pancake

*Prep time: 10 minutes | Cooking time: 40 minutes | Servings: 2*

**Ingredients:**

- 1 teaspoon apple cider vinegar
- 1 teaspoon vanilla extract
- 1 cup almond milk
- 1/3 cup almond flour
- 1 tablespoon Erythritol
- ½ teaspoon baking powder
- 1 tablespoon butter

**Directions:**

Melt the butter until liquid. Stir the almond milk in the liquid butter. Add almond flour and Erythritol. Mix up the mixture and add vanilla extract and baking powder. Add an apple cider vinegar and whisk the mixture until smooth. Pour the pancake batter in the instant pot bowl. Close and seal the instant pot lid. Set the "Manual" mode for 40 minutes. When the time is over – let the pancake chill a little bit and then transfer it onto the serving plate.

**Nutrition value/serving:** calories 433, fat 43.1, fiber 4.5, carbs 10.9, protein 6.1

# Conclusion

While reading the last pages of this cookbook you have already known an enormous amount of delicious Keto diet meals that you can easily cook every day. Instant pot is really miracle invention of Canadian designer Rober Wang. During the years it has been developing and changing. Nowadays, this super multi-cooker can help you with cooking almost all meals – from long-time stewing to making tasty and healthy yogurts.

Instant pot has been experiencing absolutely success all over the world. You can hardly find the house where there is no instant pot.

There are different types of the instant pot and its capabilities depend on the model you buy. Nevertheless, there are basic programs that are present in every model. Such programs are slow cooker and rice cooker, steamer and pressure cooker (LOW/HIGH pressure), saute, yogurt making and warmer.

There are a lot of improved cookers that include cake and egg maker. Some appliances allow sterilizing inside them.

Which dish is better to use in Instant Pot?

You can use almost all ceramic and glass dishes. If there are any restrictions about dishes – you will find them in the recipe. Besides it, you can find special dishes and accessories exactly for Instant Pot. Supermarkets and online shops suggest a great deal of special appliance such as spoons, tray, ladders, molds, springform pans, pot holders, etc. All these tools can make the process of cooking simpler and faster.

The essential point is the choice of the size of the dishes. It should match the size of your Instant Pot. Otherwise, you risk getting burned or injured while cooking.

Instant Pot has fundamentally reversed the idea of cooking time. Now cooking will take a few minutes and for complex dishes an hour or two. The instant Pot makes magic things in comparison with the ordinary cooking method that takes hours to cook the dinner.

The perfect combo of the Instant Pot and this cookbook will inspire to bring to life your new culinary masterpieces and follow the Keto diet easily and effectively for your health.

# Recipe index

## BROCCOLI
Coconut Milk Broccoli, 42
Broccoli Mash, 44

## CABBAGE
Curry Cabbage, 38
Cabbage Petals, 41

## CARROTS
Shredded Pot Roast, 49
Juicy Chopped Pork, 56
Carrot Cake Cups, 62

## CAULIFLOWER
Cauliflower Cream Soup, 22
Tender Mashed Cauliflower, 34
Tender Cauliflower Florets, 37
Hash Brown, 41
Cauliflower Rice, 43

## CELERY
Breakfast Chicken Hash, 18
Celery Ragout, 36
Stuffed Celery Stalks with Goat
Cheese, 42

## CHEDDAR CHEESE
Cheese Omelet, 14
Stuffed Mushrooms with Cheese, 28

## CHICKEN
Breakfast Meatballs, 9
Tender Chicken Breast with Coconut
Milk, 9
Morning Burrito Bowl, 10
Chicken Rolls, 13
Keto Breakfast Sandwich, 18
Breakfast Chicken Hash, 18
Eggplant Kebob, 20
Buffalo Chicken Soup, 25
Greek-Style Chicken Thighs, 25
Chicken Stew with Mushrooms, 27
Zucchini Salad, 29
Garam Masala, 31
Rosemary Chicken Wings, 33
Chicken Tikka Masala, 47
Chicken Adobo, 48
Stuffed Chicken Breast, 51
Buffalo Chicken, 52
Spicy Chicken Drumsticks, 53
Chicken Kebab with Green Pepper, 55
Parmesan Chicken Cubes, 55

## CHOCOLATE
Brownie in Cup, 60
Keto Brownies, 64
Chocolate Cake, 67
Lava Cake, 68
Keto Hot Chocolate, 71

## COCONUT
Breakfast Porridge, 15

## COCONUT FLAKES
Coconut Bites, 61
Soft Keto Cheesecake, 62
Coconut Bars, 71

## COCONUT FLOUR
Bacon Muffins, 16
Lemon Cakes in a Mug, 69

**COCONUT MILK**
Tender Chicken Breast with Coconut Milk, 9
Coconut Milk Prawns, 19
Fabulous Seabass Steak, 29
Garam Masala, 31
Lamb Stew, 32
Tender Mashed Cauliflower, 34
Coconut Milk Broccoli, 42
Shrimp Soup, 50
Pudding Cake, 65

**COURFETTE**
Spicy Courgette Zoodles, 34

**CREAM**
Butter Prawns, 26
Bacon Chowder, 26
Spicy Chicken Drumsticks, 53
Cream Pork Liver, 58
Garlic Beef Stew, 59
Pumpkin Pie Pudding, 60
Keto Mousse, 61
Soft Keto Cheesecake, 62
Crème Brulee, 63

**CREAM CHEESE**
Egg Cups, 11
Pumpkin Cheesecake, 68

**CUCUMBERS**
Morning Burrito Bowl, 10
Zucchini Salad, 29

**EGGPLANTS**
Eggplant Kebob, 20
Meatball Stew, 23

Eggplants Stew, 39
Stuffed Eggplants, 58

**EGGS**
Soft-Boiled Eggs, 8
Spinach Frittata, 8
Breakfast Meatballs, 9
Crunchy Bacon Strips, 10
Breakfast Casserole, 11
Egg Cups, 11
Morning Cups, 12
Quiche, 12
Stuffed Eggs with Bacon, 13
Egg Bites, 14
Cheese Omelet, 14
Light Stuffed Green Peppers, 16
Creamy Boiled Eggs, 17
Salmon Quiche, 30
Egg Salad, 45
Salmon Cutlets, 54
Spicy Meatloaf, 57
Pumpkin Pie Pudding, 60
Brownie in Cup, 60
Coconut Bites, 61
Keto Mousse, 61
Carrot Cake Cups, 62
Crème Brulee, 63
Blackberry Muffins, 63
Lemon Curd, 64
Mug Cake, 65
Cardamom Tender Cake, 66
Cinnamon Roll, 67
Lava Cake, 68
Custard Cups, 69

**FENNEL**
Roasted Fennel Salad, 43

**FETA**
Kale-Feta Saute 40

**FISH**
Tuna Casserole, 28
Fabulous Seabass Steak, 29
Fish Cakes, 30
Seabass with Parmesan, 57

**GOAT CHEESE**
Stuffed Celery Stalks with Goat
Cheese, 42

**GREEN BEANS**
Butter Green Beans, 38

**GREEN PEPPERS**
Light Stuffed Green Peppers, 16
Keto Stuffed Peppers, 21
Chicken Kebab with Green Pepper, 55

**KALE**
Tender Kale, 39
Kale-Feta Saute, 40

**LAMB**
Lamb Stew, 32

**LEMON**
Lemon Salmon Fillet, 19
Greek-Style Chicken Thighs, 25
Lemon Curd, 64
Lemon Cakes in a Mug, 69

**LETTUCE**
Creamy Boiled Eggs, 17
Keto Breakfast Sandwich, 18
Thyme Salmon Salad, 45

Egg Salad, 45

**MUSHROOMS**
Chicken Stew with Mushrooms, 27
Stuffed Mushrooms with Cheese, 28
Lamb Stew, 32
White Mushrooms Saute, 35
Beef Stew, 50
Beef Stroganoff, 53

**NOODLES**
Asian Noodles, 44

**ONION**
Pork Bites, 15
Keto Breakfast Sandwich, 18
Breakfast Chicken Hash, 18
Shredded Beef, 22
Basil Beef Ribs, 24
Mongolian Beef, 27
Asian Meatballs, 32
Eggplants Stew, 39
Chicken Tikka Masala, 47
Butter Beef, 56
Spicy Meatloaf, 57

**PARMESAN**
Breakfast Casserole, 11
Quiche, 12
Egg Bites, 14
Light Stuffed Green Peppers, 16
Lasagna with Zucchini, 21
Cauliflower Cream Soup, 22
Buffalo Chicken Soup, 25
Tuna Casserole, 28
Fragrant Asparagus, 37
Eggplants Stew, 39

Hash Brown, 41
Zucchini Boats with Cheese, 46
Parmesan Chicken Cubes, 55
Seabass with Parmesan, 57

**PARSLEY**
Butter Green Beans, 38
Roasted Fennel Salad, 43

**PECANS**
Sauteed Spinach, 36

**PORK**
Pork Bites, 15
Asian Meatballs, 31
Pulled Pork, 32
Chili Verde, 47
Pork Carnitas, 52
Pork Chops, 54
Juicy Chopped Pork, 56
Cream Pork Liver, 58
Stuffed Eggplants, 58

**PUMPKIN**
Pumpkin Pie Pudding, 60
Pumpkin Cheesecake, 68

**SALMON**
Lemon Salmon Fillet, 19
Garlic Salmon, 23
Salmon Quiche, 30
Thyme Salmon Salad, 45
Salmon Cutlets, 54

**SALSA**
Chili Verde, 47

**SEAFOOD**
Quiche, 12
Coconut Milk Prawns, 19
Butter Prawns, 26

**SHRIMPS**
Stuffed Avocado Boats, 17
Shrimp Soup, 50

**SPINACH**
Spinach Frittata, 8
Morning Cups, 12
Celery Ragout, 36
Sauteed Spinach, 36

**TOFU**
Kale-Feta Saute 40

**TOMATOES**
Breakfast Casserole, 11
Ropa Vieja, 24
Fragrant Taco Meat, 49
Keto Chili, 51

**ZUCCHINI**
Lasagna with Zucchini, 21
Zucchini Salad, 29
Zucchini Zoodles with Chili Pepper, 35
Zucchini Boats with Cheese, 46
Keto Apple-Free Crisps, 70

Made in the USA
Lexington, KY
11 June 2019